BECOMING THE STORY

The Power of PREhab™

By

Loriana Hernandez-Aldama

BECOMING THE STORY

The Power of PREhab™

By

Loriana Hernandez-Aldama

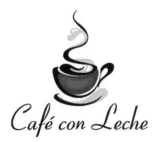

Café con Leche

Becoming the Story: The Power of PREhab™

© Copyright 2021, Loriana Hernandez-Aldama

ISBN 978-1-7370614-0-3

Cover Design By: Drex Earle of Bounce Marketing

Pit Crew Image (page 75) by Skeeze from Pixabay

Published by

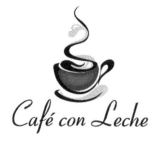

Café con Leche

3 Griffin Hill Court
The Woodlands, TX. 77382
281-465-0119
www.savvyliterary.com
www.cafeconlechebooks.com

Contents

Dedication

To all my cancer warriors, ArmorUp for LIFE®,
stay prepared, we are in this together!

To those we have lost, your silence is deafening.
I miss you. I hear you. Every. Single. Day.
I will never stop fighting for you.

May this book be the voice for those too tired to speak,
those no longer with us and those who may one day
walk this same journey.

Together we can improve the patient experience, boost
patient compliance and outcomes and diversify enrollment
for clinical trials for the greater good.

******

To my husband Cesar:

You are the calm in every storm. The love of my life. The epitome of crisis management. When you said "I do" and said, "In sickness and in health" you didn't know for years it would be more sickness than health. You stood by me. You slept next to me. You never wavered. You are my ROCK. I love you.

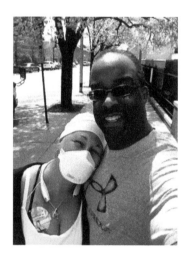 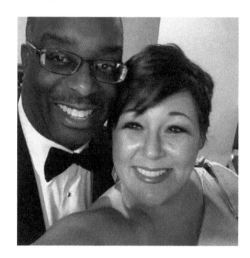

To my son Gabriel:

When I kissed you goodbye for the first fight of my life, I didn't know if it would be my last. I'm so blessed and honored to watch you grow up. You are my world. Every step I took. Every tear I cried. Every obstacle I faced, I heard your voice saying "Mami Mami" and I found strength. I love you with all my heart and all my soul. Today and every day. You are the reason I ArmorUp for LIFE® from the minute I wake up until I go to sleep. I love you.

To my sister Lisa, My HERO:

You gave me the gift of LIFE. The gift of a second chance. The gift of time. Thank you!
Thank you for your life saving bone marrow. Thank you for the privilege to watch my son grow up. Thank you for giving my son his mother back and my husband his wife back. Now, I am you. I have your DNA. We are ONE. Love you!!

To my Mom, Barbara:

Thank you for raising my son for an entire year so I could fight for my life. You are my hero. While raising your two-year-old grandson was more than you ever expected to do at the age of 70, you formed a bond with Gabriel he will never forget. Thank you for your unconditional love and support.

To my Dad, Al and Stepmom Jane:

Thank you for stepping in and helping my mom raise Gabriel during my fight and also taking in my fur child, Isabella and treating her like your own. I'm blessed to have your unconditional love and unwavering support.

Acknowledgements

You can't fight this war alone. I certainly didn't.
I still ask for help.

From coast to coast, I was surrounded by
incredible heroes and angels who shared their many gifts to
help me find my voice and my purpose. The long list should
serve as a reminder to everyone on this journey that you
MUST ask for help.

Look at this pit crew. There are many more than
I had room to list.

Each person played a role in my survival.

Each person helped in some way successfully lead me to the
finish line and into survivorship, through the depression,
PTSD, another cancer and more surgeries so
I could survive and thrive.

The length of this list speaks volumes.

If you ever thought you didn't have a gift to offer to a
cancer patient, think again.

100% of the proceeds of this book will go back to ArmorUp
for LIFE® so we can help more patients.

To all the warriors:

Those heroes I lost on my hall like Paul, Ryan and many others, I will forever be your voice.

To the heroes who I fought alongside and survived, we must lift up our voices for those who may walk the path we once walked.

Maria Dennis, Jenn Aparacio, Barb Cavelius and others, we are ONE community.

To my "Pit Crew" who helped successfully get me to the finish line.

HEROES on the front lines, I love you. I'm grateful for you.

RESEARCHERS: Thank you for your passion, your relentless search for answers for patients like me and countless others. We need you. We are counting on you.

Doctors:

- Dr. Mark Levis, Johns Hopkins Leukemia Oncologist and his entire team
- Dr. Brian Druker, Knight Cancer Institute
- Dr. Robin Avery- Johns Hopkins, Infectious Disease
- Dr. David Steensma-Dana Farber Institute
- Dr. Azar- Johns Hopkins Immunologist
- Dr. Shar Kavoussi, my fertility doctor who gave me the gift of my son Gabriel and cried as he told me, "You can't have another baby, you have cancer."
- Dr. Katherine Steele, Penn Medicine, Medical Dermatology
- Dr. Kathleen Murphy, Penn Medicine, Infectious Disease

- Dr. Allison Chase - FOX contributor who helped me psychologically during my treatment because I didn't have the support I needed at the hospital.

Physician Assistant

- Jackie Jung

Nurses:

- Rita Stella
- Annlise Calypso
- Robinah Campbell
- Kristy Hildebrandt-Chaney
- Brynn Puller
- Deborah Henry
- Carolina Hickman
- Julia Schuster
- Leah Chandler
- Laura Clayton
- Rita Stella
- Mikki Jackels
- Genny Dalton
- Susannah Dowling

To my friend Alice Alston. Thank you!

Thank you for jumping into action and launching a campaign to share my story and raise money so we could focus on the fight and not our finances. The financial toxicity of cancer is overlooked. It is a reality. Alice, without you spearheading our support, we would have lost our home.

A special thank you to my FOX 7 News Director Pam Vaught, who played a big role in saving my life. She allowed me to file reports from my bedside for a year. She gave me purpose. She made me feel empowered when I wanted to give up. Through my storytelling and belief my message would save lives, I felt compelled to fight and an obligation not to give up despite my strength saying otherwise.

My FOX Family who believed in me and gave me HOPE

- Pam Vaught
- Dave Froehlich
- Zack Shields
- Lauren Petrowski
- Jenni Lee
- Scott Fisher
- Stacey Davis
- Noelle Newton
- Aly Kerr
- Crysta Lee
- Josh Lippold
- Maureen Conway
- Dr. Manny Alvarez

Our Media Family and Friends—

- Princell Hair
- Anzio Williams
- Anne-Marie Green
- Julie Donaldson
- Chick Hernandez
- Cristina Hernandez
- Eric Schuster
- Andy & Janice Ockerhausen
- Joe & Tracey Garcia
- Rebecca Miller
- Manel Coleau

To my incredible friends who despite their own demanding careers and obligations and took time to create, brand and launch ArmorUp for LIFE® while I was in the midst of my fight. I'm in awe of your kindness. You believed in me, believed in my message and gave me purpose.

- Drex Earle
- Jason Stanford
- Amy Katzenberg

To those who believed in me, believed in my story and gave me a platform to amplify the patient voice and change the patient experience:

- Rob Ruckman
- Amanda DePalma
- Jasmine Healy
- Alex Cherry
- Jan Nissen
- Sophia Nelson
- Melissa Rauscher-Ludwig
- Kristine Illaria
- Kristin Roosevelt
- Dr. Lou DeGennaro
- Marcie Klein
- Nancy Terry
- Andrea Greif
- Jonathon Wilson
- James Roberts
- Liz Wolf
- Nancy Hubacher
- Leo Tucker
- Natali Ceniza
- Janice Caprelian
- Stephanie Lee
- Rum Ngo
- Kristin Staples
- Megan Imbert
- Nicole Anderson
- Elaine Grobman
- Tina Johnson
- Katie Nelson
- Ryan Huss
- Tara Haarlander
- Amber Summers
- Jeff Livick
- Kevin Chadwick
- Jamie Graham
- Inga Koeppe
- Vicki Bodwell
- Dillar Schwartz
- Debijo Wheatley
- Dr. Haress Rahim
- Lisa Regoni
- Katie Nelson
- Donna Christou

To those friends who took care of me, bathed me, fed me, thank you!

- Tracey & Joe Garcia
- Jo-Ann Carricate
- Tracy Ganske
- Deepthi Chithajallu
- Miranda & Robert Whitcher

Those who gave of themselves so I make memories with my family and also save my strength... Thank you! Thank you for endless help... the groceries, the meals, the fitness gear, the flowers, the prayers, the meditation, watching/caring for Gabriel and even caring for our fur child "Coco." We could not have done this without you.

- Beatriz Torrente
- Craig Piatti
- Kristi & Eddie Rodriguez
- Christopher Nastasi
- Joanne Nastasi
- Donna Christou
- Janice & John Perez
- Rick Huss & Christy Grossini
- Lorraine Kayser & Shawn Bradley
- Misty Cebry
- Maryann Crittendon
- Chanelle Bishop
- Jo-Ann Carricarte
- Kerry & Henry Willie
- Megan Imbert
- Debijo Wheatley
- Kelly Yiadom
- Paul and Terri Finneran
- Tracey Detwiler Robinson
- Karen Benbatoul
- Rebecca Miller
- Beth & Adam Prius
- Jinal Patel
- Janine Portner
- Rohan Menon
- Lisa Salladino
- Sarah Bender
- Tracey Parent

- Matt Ouano
- Marylin Mallo
- Art Acevedo
- Rick, Natalie, Ashley Torrente
- Jose Torrente
- Jorge Gomez
- Muggeo family
- Courtney Osman
- Melissa Ayers
- Lisa Buenaventura Rice
- Foti Kallergis
- Maryann Crittendon
- Jane & David Muggeo
- Thad & Jennifer Walker
- Teresa S. Yasutis
- Jeanise & Luis Rosado
- Vicki, Tanner and Lauren Brooks
- Becca Moreno
- Nisha Azad
- Maria Velasquez
- Nicole Carswell
- Laura Arias & Jessica Lacour
- Jessica Smith
- Deanna Cain
- Neha Oberoi
- Kelly Yiadom

To the warriors (survivors) who showed up to unpack our VA house while I fought for my life before even meeting me— Thank you!

- Jamie Tinschert - you are amazing.

To my spiritual pit crew members—thank you for the countless FaceTime prayer sessions and free meditation and yoga when cancer was breaking me down and I was ready to give up. Each of you lifted me up.

- Todd & Valerie Wallace
- Azi Tavassoli

Leukemia & Lymphoma Society

- Dr. Lou DeGennaro
- Marcie Klein
- Dr. Gwen Nichols
- Andrea Greif
- Ria Freiberg
- Beth Gorman
- Amanda Tiede
- Jaclyn Toll
- Kate Kusarak

To the non-profits funding breakthrough treatments-Thank you!

The Leukemia & Lymphoma Society

Thank you for your tireless efforts, your BEAT AML Trial, the researchers to advance breakthrough treatments. I am grateful.

American Association of Cancer Research (AACR)

American Cancer Society

Susan G. Komen

Foreword

Some people think in words. I think in images. It happens after decades of working as an anchor and reporter in television news. A story doesn't make it on the nightly news unless there are compelling pictures to go with it. The old line in the TV business goes . . . "without pictures it's called radio." The thing is a picture or image only ever represents a fleeting moment in a story. This book tells the part of Loriana's story that you would not have seen in the flickering images on the evening news. The part of the story that taught her life lessons worth passing on.

Speaking of images, when I think of Loriana, the image that comes to mind is a supernova. She has the brilliance and illumination of a star. She is warm, exciting with what seems like boundless energy. I'm no NASA scientist so I'll keep it simple. As I understand it, the thing about a supernova is that it is held together by pressure. Gravity is pushing down and the star's energy is pushing out, keeping the structure intact. But once the energy diminishes, gravity wins out, and the star collapses. Sometimes people collapse too. Lori's world collapsed with a cancer diagnosis. She was married to a supportive man, had a successful career, became a mother and was preparing for baby number two. Her life imploded but she would not. Instead, she would stop wearing exhaustion as a badge of honor and start wearing armor. She would "ArmorUp" for the battles ahead and now you can too.

There may have been times when you felt like the pressure was building toward a collapse. I had a collapsed of my own . . . quite literally. I had a fever and chills and passed out at the anchor desk at the beginning of a show. Not wanting to let my crew down, I didn't dare call out sick. I honestly thought I could push through it. I mistakenly thought it would be hard to replace me. Within minutes a fill-in anchor was at the desk and finished the show. I'm saying this with a chuckle, though it was scary at the time. An embarrassing reminder that the show will always go on without you . . . but it will also be there when you come back. Especially if you come back stronger, healthier, happier.

This book is a reminder and a guide. Take it easy on yourself, take care of yourself, take the warning signs seriously. The signs are friendly reminders that unlike supernovas, people don't have to burn out to shine bright.

Love yourself and each other.

—Anne-Marie Green, Network News Correspondent and Anchor

Introduction

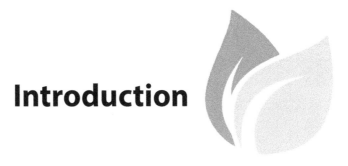

A man is walking down the street and falls into a hole so deep he can't climb out. He yells for help until a doctor comes along.

"Doctor, can you help me?"

The doctor writes out a prescription and throws it into the hole and walks away. Same with the priest who comes by after more caterwauling: He writes out a prayer and drops it into the hole with the man who is now getting increasingly desperate.

***

A few years ago, back when the stakes of political discourse often revolved around Barack Obama wearing a tan suit and whether Mitt Romney laughed authentically, I became a pundit. This was a conscious choice. I was young, and though I needed the money, I did this for free.

Punditry, to me, was a chance for me to stick up for my side. Often what we argued over were matters of state—whether the missiles were well-intended, the merits of helping the poor, the pros and cons of procreative rights—but the consequences of argument were scored in points made and defended. Did I win?

Was I right? And though I argued about important things and never argued a position I thought dishonest, I nevertheless considered the whole thing a sport to be won.

Digital evidence of this period constitutes the permanent record they so often threatened us with in school, and if you look (I do not recommend it) you will find breadcrumbs of syndicated columns scattered in local newspapers across the country, posted on websites for national publications and my local daily newspaper, and on the website of a certain national cable network. For a few years, I put in a lot of work for little money and even less effect.

But my most regular post was on a tall chair in the downtown Austin studio of the local Fox affiliate where, much like Ralph Wolf and Sam Sheepdog in the Looney Tunes cartoons, friends of mine from the opposing party would suit up, mic up, and do our best to make the other look stupid for the entertainment of those watching their local nightly news.

Often as not, the one asking me well-informed questions was Loriana Hernandez, whose book you're holding now. At the time, she was "just" a news anchor, and she took our sport seriously. She genuinely wanted her viewers to know what local political insiders such as myself and whatever able debate partner I had that day thought about the big political issue of the day. And invariably, my pretense at cynical gamesmanship would crumble in the face of her earnest questioning, and I'd end up just answering the damn question honestly, just like they teach you not to do in media training.

Two things happened about the same time: I realized that punditry is an empty enterprise that demeans our democratic experiment, and Loriana very nearly damn died. Both of us, separately, concurrently, and coincidentally, began to seek meaning, me in communication and her in suffering.

From afar, over social media, I saw her start **ArmorUp for LIFE®** Time is undefeated, and tragedy and trail alike come to us all. Loriana had come back from the suburbs of hell to warn us that fate cannot be avoided, only prepared for. ArmorUp was not some cheerful aphorism. It was an instruction. I bought a T-shirt and started doing push-ups. She had broadcast her call to arms into the world; I had answered with a weak signal on a radio she was building alone.

She reached out to ask a favor. Could I help her write a speech? Someone had asked her to talk about her experiences, and she wanted to tell them what they didn't know. I've written speeches for C-suite executives, elected officials, and the occasional object of scandal, so how hard could it be to help Loriana tell her story?

How hard can it be?

How hard can it be to help someone get a roomful of strangers to optimistically face their mortality? How hard can it be to help someone persuade healthy people to take practical steps to prepare for sickness? She told me about chemo bags and a son she couldn't see, about what it feels like to lose compatriots on the cancer ward and fight your way out.

How do you tell this story honestly without irony? How do you press your face against that window and look right at the thing to see it clearly? This was a lot harder than arguing about tan suits.

This book is like its author—a triumph. Loriana Hernandez is proof that sincerity is the new punk.

***

You are the one in the hole, yelling for help. Your friend Loriana comes by, sees the predicament you are in, and jumps into the hole with you.

"What's the big idea?" you ask. "Now there are two people in here!"

"Yes," she says, "but I've been here before, and I know the way out."

***

Some day you will find yourself in a deep hole, and you'll think of this moment right now, you reading this sentence—yes you! Right now, you have a choice to make: Do you want to know the way out?

—Jason Stanford, is an Austin-based writer whose bylines have appeared in *Texas Monthly*, the *Texas Tribune*, *Texas Highways*, the *Texas Observer*, as well as many publications that have nothing whatsoever to do with Texas. He publishes a Substack newsletter called *The Experiment*.

Preface

My heart is racing as I pace the kitchen while trying to do e-learning with my eight-year-old son Gabriel. A COVID-19 team from Penn Medicine is about to pull up and test me for the virus, and I can't focus.

"Mom, what are you worried about?" Gabriel yells at me. "You have been through worse things! Needles and biopsies in your butt. This is nothing. You are a SURVIVOR! I will cheer you on."

Well, it wasn't exactly the butt but rather the hip for countless bone marrow biopsies, but Gabriel's point stands. From afar, he witnessed my year-long battle with AML leukemia and the collateral damage that followed. If I tested positive for the virus, I knew I was ready, because I've been a veteran of this war long before it ever started.

I remember the day I said goodbye to him. As I boarded a plane for Johns Hopkins, cries of "Mommy! Mommy!" echoed down the jetway. I didn't know if I would ever see him again.

I remember the FaceTime calls as I sobbed when he asked, "How many more sleeps?" and I had no answer.

I remember being reunited with him in the lobby of Johns Hopkin, except that so much time had passed that he walked past me like we'd never met.

I remember coming home after winning my battle and realizing that sometimes, even when you win, you lose. I lost my identity. I lost my mind. My career unraveled. We were flat-broke. Heck, I was broken. I didn't know whether to make resumes in case I lived or memories in case I died.

I lost nearly everything, from my successful journalism career to my identity, *including my DNA*. Yep. You got that right. My DNA. Because of the bone marrow that I received from my sister, my body now contains her DNA, not mine. I'm not even me anymore. It's like the scene out of *Alice in Wonderland* where Alice asks, "Who in the world am I? Ah, that's the great puzzle." That's me. A great puzzle. Draw my blood and the results will tell you that there is "NO EVIDENCE of patient." No evidence. No sign of me. I can assure you, after surviving AML Leukemia followed by a bone marrow transplant and then ending up in a mind and body I no longer recognize, who I am is not who I was. I had to mourn the person I once was before I could accept my "new normal." I cringe when I hear that term now.

The good news is, isn't that what we're all going through? Been there. Done that. And I'm here for you. I know the drill. I know isolation. I know droplet precautions. Protective yellow gowns. I know germ warfare. I know loneliness. I know PTSD. Anxiety. Depression. I know suicidal thoughts. I know loss at every level. I know separation from loved ones. I know staring death in the face. I know what it is like to beat the odds. I know how to overcome.

I am a former news anchor and medical reporter who found herself on the other side of healthcare. Here's what I learned you need to know. It is my breaking news. Preparation matters.

On the fifth anniversary of surviving leukemia, we held a "Christmas in October" tree-lighting ceremony to celebrate the day, five years before, when doctors told me to go home and put up my Christmas tree early and take pictures with my son so he would have memories with me in case I died. Five years was a major milestone. Doctors predicted I had a 25 percent chance to live to see my son turn seven. Living to this day was a huge deal.

Then came the most unexpected gift . . . breast cancer. The trade-off, I was told, likely caused by the full-body radiation used to save my life.

It was time for me to go to war again.

A high-risk double mastectomy for a patient without her own DNA and a history of rejecting blood transfusions earned me a special designation. My Johns Hopkins leukemia oncologist called me N1 . . . for being his first patient to go from a liquid cancer to a solid tumor. It had to happen to someone. I drew the short straw and fought it head-on. Again, I was prepared. And again, cancer stole yet another piece of my identity: my breasts, the ones that once fed and nourished my son. Gone. In an instant. The losses piled up.

I *survived* again, but this time it happened during the COVID-19 pandemic. When the world went into a time-out, so did my treatment and follow-up appointments. Cancer wasn't cancelled, but it sure felt like it. My life was once again in limbo. My husband went from spouse to home healthcare nurse and had to start packing my wounds left over from the surgery.

I survived. I thrived. I won. AGAIN.

Now with COVID-19 taking center stage, sure, there is an element of fear. I don't want to go back "there" again. But as others panic, I feel a strange sense of calm. I've been here before, and I'm ready. My leukemia battle prepared me for *this* moment. I think others struggling right now can pull strength from survivors like myself. We've been there. Done that. Physically. Mentally. Emotionally, Spiritually . . . *financially.*

I lost a lot, but what I gained is what I want to share with all of you. My pivot became my purpose. I discovered the biggest breaking story of my career, and I need to share it with you. You must prepare, because something will come. The more fit you are going into the fight of your life, the better you will get through it. I learned this through each cancer battle, and we are learning this with COVID-19, too.

I call this ArmoringUp for LIFE®.

We all need to ArmorUp, not just physically but emotionally and mentally, because now we are all in the cancer ward. No one is immune, and humanity is the marker. How you prehabilitate and prepare will determine if you survive. You must prepare mentally for the fight, physically for the suffering, and spiritually for the strength. Many of us feel a lack of control, but what you can control is preparation: what you eat, how much you exercise, the stress and toxicity in your life, how much deep restorative sleep you get, your spiritual and financial preparation. The choice is yours.

As we all look over our shoulders fearing COVID-19, let's not forget other illnesses are waiting in the wings and we can't let our guards down.

Cancer isn't cancelled, heart disease isn't cancelled, your next illness isn't cancelled.

The time is now to start preparing your body for illness. You have the power today to become your own hero by preparing today for whatever comes your way tomorrow. Remember, surviving is a job. It's now my only job.

Make it yours.

[By the way, I tested negative!]

CHAPTER 1

The Wake-Up Call

Never be Complacent

Even if you think you have it all, your life can flip in an instant. The news never stopped, and neither did I. For more than two decades in TV broadcasting, I'd had many wake-up calls in the middle of the night, for all sorts of breaking developments and tragic events that would soon become headlines. Earthquakes. Tornadoes. SWAT Stand-offs. Wildfires and political chaos. I would be awakened into a sweat to scramble out the door and be first on the air and share the stories of loss and devastation. With each disaster, my heart would ache as family members fell to their knees in disbelief. For natural disasters, I would carefully walk over debris left of what once was, as families literally picked up the pieces of their lives and cried out "what is next?" I was there to listen, gather information, and tell their story. I heard their pain, thought I felt their pain, and even carried it in my heart with me, but at the end of the day I would go back to my life, untouched by the crisis. I would get to my own reality of award-winning anchor, medical and

1

fitness reporter, burning the candle at both ends to get the story. I worked hard. I played hard. That reality meant returning to the galas and glamour of a high-profile news anchor to raise money for wonderful causes for people who needed help.

It made me feel good and justified the glitz and glamour.

Plus, I never needed help.

Nope.

I was invincible.

But in November of 2013, I got the kind of wake-up call I never expected.

Suddenly, the tables were turned. My world flipped upside-down and I found myself on the other side of healthcare . . . needing the very help I helped fund.

> Much like that feeling when COVID-19 woke up the world. We were all caught off guard. But long before COVID, my life as I knew it flipped upside down and unraveled in ways I never imagined.
>
> I was about to enlist in a war I didn't want to sign up for, including a germ warfare that would change my life forever.

I was lying in bed at midnight, and as usual my alarm was set to go off at 1:45 AM so I could get ready for another day at my dream job, anchoring the FOX network's morning show in Austin, Texas. Suddenly, I was jolted by a horrific pain, like someone was stabbing me or breaking my bones in half. I clutched my right arm, sat up in a panic and screamed at the top of my lungs.

But no one heard me: My husband was away, working on the East Coast, and our twenty-month-old son, Gabriel, was (somehow) sound asleep next to me. The shooting pain wouldn't let up. In the dark I managed to stumble down the stairs, screaming "Oh my God. Oh my God." I grabbed an ice pack from the freezer and phoned Cesar in Maryland.

"Slow down and catch your breath," he urged, over and over. "Tell me what's going on."

I had no idea what was going on, and I couldn't stop sobbing. The ache was bizarre, like a truck had just parked on my arm.

My mind started to race for an explanation. Had I hurt myself lifting weights at the gym in "boot camp"? Did I overstretch in my hot yoga class? Could this be a return of the shingles that had broken out during pregnancy?

Whatever the cause, I had no time to puzzle over it. I couldn't go to an emergency room to get it checked out; it was nearly time to head in to anchor our five-hour Fox morning news show. The news wouldn't wait, so my health crisis had to. "Be tough and stick it out" is how I'd built my career from the very beginning, and I wasn't about to change tactics.

It was pointless trying to sleep anymore. I pulled on my clothes, packed ice on my arm, and drove to the station. In pain, I got out my flat iron and got my hair TV ready as I sobbed. I still had to look the part. Pain wasn't an excuse to not look TV ready.

Of course, I'd go to work. After all, *my colleagues needed me!* Isn't that what we all say? And at 2 AM, I couldn't call just anybody to fill in. I couldn't leave my co-anchors, Dave Froelich and Lauren Petrowski hanging. We were a team. We were in the middle of a crucial ratings period. Plus, I *had* to finish my special report for the national network's health and medical coverage.

It is an unspoken rule in the news business that, unless you're pretty much dead, you just don't call in sick during ratings sweeps or when there are on-going developing stories making national headlines. In twenty years on TV, I'd had to miss only one—when I took a brief medical leave for Gabriel's birth. In fact, any time an unexpected absence was announced at an editorial meeting, a chill would descend over the conference room. "Ohhh, okay then," people would mutter, and "Hmmm." I was not about to be that person. It's my policy never to quit anything. I push through it. That's been my lifelong MO, and my message day in and day out as a medical and fitness reporter.

I *especially* didn't want a fill-in taking *my* chair at the anchor desk. If anybody was going to get good ratings in *my* time slot, it was going to be me. As TV talent, you always know in the back of your mind that you can be replaced easily enough by someone younger, thinner, and cheaper. Cesar has worked for various networks at a management level and I'd heard the conversations over the years about anchors in other markets being pushed aside. I had seen it happen myself. In fact, *I* was the replacement when, at an early age, I got my on-air break!

The newsroom is no place to show weakness. I'd show up, and I'd be *on:* alert and looking my best, fashionably on, with my hair flat ironed and high-definition makeup perfectly applied. When the little red light came on, I'd smile for the camera, no matter what.

Why? Because the show must go on. So, the nanny showed up at 3 AM. We passed like ships in the night. I hopped in my car with tears rolling down my eyes while in horrendous pain and I drove, not to a damn hospital, but to the station. My career was my world. Damnit, I was sticking to my routine. I couldn't

4

deviate from it now. And like clockwork, I rolled into work at 3:30 AM, took the steps to the second floor make up/green room (not the elevator-of course. I needed to burn a few more calories). I opened the door, turned up my Latino beats, and held *Icy Hot* on my arm. I danced my way around the green room, taking out shadows one by one out of my bag and neatly placing them all on the counter. I plugged in the flat iron, rolled out my makeup brushes, and then looked over scripts one by one so I could prepare for the back-to-back interviews of guests on our morning show. Between trying to glamorize myself and get familiar with each and every guest on schedule for the day, my mind was racing that something wasn't right. But I kept going. Next up, opening my lunch cooler, taking out my needle and injecting fertility hormones into my stomach. I was also preparing to be a mom again. Remember, I was invincible? Oh, did I mention, I was still in pain? Mind over matter. I'm good at that. I compartmentalized that pain and focused on my work, preparing for interview after interview. Made grammatical corrections to scripts and forged ahead.

I ignored EVERY SINGLE WARNING SIGN, including this obvious one.

Then it was SHOWTIME.

The lights came up, the sign flashed and I was "ON".

Four-thirty AM. . . . And 3. . . 2. . . 1. . .

"Rise and shine everyone, thanks for waking up with us on Fox 7 on this gorgeous day here in Austin. We'll take a look at traffic and weather. Then after the headlines it's time again for me to help you transform your diet in my segment Clean Eating, *bringing you*

amazing meals of yummy nutrient-dense food that can help fight cancer. We are back in just a moment . . ."

But that day, during the breaks between sound bites, when they killed the lights so we wouldn't sweat off our makeup, I madly smeared *Icy Hot* cream on my arm. I alternated with ice packs and tried to make a joke out of my predicament to Dave while we were on the set. I ground my teeth against the pain, but when the lights returned, I sat up, smiled, and carried on like nothing was wrong.

Somehow, I hung in and anchored for five and a half hours, then finished my reporting work. I got the nanny to stay late with Gabriel so I could drive straight to my massage therapist, thinking she'd be able to "fix" my bizarre pain. She did her best, but nothing worked. I went home to my sweet baby and kept up a good front.

After a few days, the pain went away completely. Whew! So, I never followed up with a doctor.

I resumed my normal routine, which consisted of long hours and precious little sleep. Gabriel was colicky, and he'd often scream until 9:30 or 10 PM. I'd "nap" from 10 PM until 1:45 AM, then rise and shine for the morning-anchor schedule. Meanwhile, my married colleagues would have handed off their kids to a spouse at 7 PM and hit the sack. I followed work with rigorous workouts at the gym or yoga, and emceeing community events, speaking at or hosting upscale galas with the who's who—all while preaching the power of a healthy lifestyle of diet and exercise to my viewers. In between, I tended to my long-distance marriage and essentially was a single mom to our toddler.

All that sacrifice, determination and effort did pay-off: I had an ambitious, supportive husband (even if Cesar's job kept him near Washington, D.C.). We were the ecstatic parents of Gabriel—and working to get pregnant with our second child. I had friendships, a good salary that allowed us to help support other family members, and work I loved in one of the most amazing cities ever, Austin, Texas, where I would call home for ten years.

I was the clean-eating, green-drinking yoga enthusiast. Host of a "Clean Eating" show to teach everyone how to transform their lives through diet and exercise. I was fit and healthy, secure and *invincible*.

I thought I had it all.

And then I didn't.

I went from telling everyone's story to *"Becoming the Story."*

I also had cancer, running through the blood in my veins.

My OB-GYN physician stumbled upon the evidence. A biopsy finally confirmed the diagnosis: Acute Myeloid Leukemia (AML).

The moment I got the news, my illusion of strength and health was betrayed. The career that had so defined me began to unravel.

In less than forty-eight hours, faster than the warning we got about the shelter in place for COVID-19, I was on a plane and my then two-year-old son ripped from my arms so I could fight for my life. I looked out that window in silence and feared I would never see him again as I faced a year-long, aggressive treatment program to save my life. I would say goodbye to my angelic son, the light of my life, not knowing if I would ever see him again. Not knowing if that day together would be our last.

In fact, now when I think of those who died during the COVID pandemic and never got to see their family members again, my heart breaks into pieces. I can't even imagine the pain.

But for those who escaped COVID-19, I say this: I would have given anything to have the kind of "quarantine" we were ordered to for COVID-19. "Stay in your home, with your loved ones, stay healthy and not face death." Sign me up! Instead, this was more like, "You will not see your son for a year, you have a 25% chance of survival (if that). You will have to wear an N95 mask 24/7 because after the chemo destroys your immune system then any germ can kill you and you won't be able to fight. You will be on droplet precautions because of that, and your spouse will have to wear a yellow droplet precaution gown to see you. No touching, no holding hands. No contact. Put your head before your heart and think long- term and not short-term if you want to get out alive. It was more like "survive in here and you will have your son for a lifetime. See him now and you die."

Holy shit is right. That was the quarantine I faced. Not a quarantine to "sit on your couch" and enjoy your family.

Plans to reunite our family under one roof were dashed. Instead, I would trade the friends, fans, and colleagues of my beloved community in Texas for a hospital thousands of miles away in a strange city where I knew no one.

After two weeks of chemotherapy and radiation, I would be almost too sick and weak to keep food down or crawl across the floor to the bathroom. I had run a marathon before, and each trip from the bed to the bathroom felt like one. Existing was exhausting. Every day I would ask if I was going to die. Bearing a second child was out of the question.

Soon, the marriage that for years had weathered two time zones was under tremendous strain. We were breaking and I was broken—physically, financially, emotionally, and I was running on fumes spiritually.

For me, this devastation arose from cancer, as it does for millions of others each year. But such upheaval can have other origins: divorce, a death in the family, economic downturns, disabilities, or natural catastrophes. None of these are uncommon.

The lives we humans build are more fragile than we imagine.

CHAPTER 2

The Foundation

Drive and Determination

Drive and determination brought me tremendous success. They also planted the seeds for my disease.

I ignored the wake-up call that my body had sent me in November and pushed it from my mind.

You might have a warning light going off right now. Like that warning light in your car that goes on from time to time and flickers and makes your stomach sink because you simply don't have time to deal with it. You're too busy. It's not convenient. Then the light goes out and you believe the problem went away, right? And if you are reading this during the pandemic or after it, you might even question now why you never addressed it. That was me five years ago before I was diagnosed with an often-fatal form of leukemia. I ignored the warning signs. EVERY. SINGLE. ONE.

I had a year in that hospital to reflect on how I had planted the seeds for my disease by the go-go-go mentality. Each time it pointed to

> my sleep deprivation. My mantra was always, "I will sleep when I'm dead." Little did I know that lack of sleep could *leave* me dead. Plus, in the midst of climbing the ladder in my career, who had time to self-reflect? There was always another goal waiting to be accomplished. I realized . . . I'd grown used to doing that.

Actually, I'd been tired for months. Exhausted, really. *But who on earth wouldn't be?* Less than four hours of regular sleep isn't enough to sustain a new mother, let alone one with a demanding, high-profile career, and postpartum depression, and a long-distance marriage. I was running on fumes, and I thought it was normal, under the circumstances. Couldn't be a medical problem, it was "just stress."

My dad had long described my lifestyle as "putting a gallon into a quart," warning that I couldn't get away with that approach forever. "Shoehorn" was the nickname my co-anchor out in California, Rich Rodriguez, gave me. He often accused and teased me of squeezing so much into my days there was no room for rest or even a schedule change.

The previous fall season, my OB-GYN had sent me to a local oncologist just to be sure. He'd assured me I was no less healthy than most overwhelmed new mothers. "Not you—you are the fitness guru," he observed. "You are just run down from a busy schedule. You are fine. Go home and enjoy your baby and enjoy life."

So later on, when the screaming pain seared my arm in the middle of the night, I clung to my denial.

All the warning lights were going off. My gut feeling was saying something was wrong, but how?

Remember, *I was invincible.*

From the outside looking in, my life looked crazy. I had a high-profile job. I was scrambling around the clock as a working, single parent with a 3 AM call for a nanny to show up daily to watch our then two-year-old son. We only saw Cesar for about forty-eight hours twice a month—when one of us would fly across the country for an abbreviated "weekend" visit. Something had to give, but *no way* was I going to give up the career I had worked so hard to build, to ultimately lose my identity. As it turned out, it was the very thing I ended up losing anyway. But I also knew deep down something wasn't right. How long could I physically go on burning the candle at both ends trying to "have it all"?

> I was living in a world of wants, not needs, like many are guilty of doing. Cancer changed that for me. Cancer or COVID may have changed this for you.

I also wanted another baby. Why not add that to the stress and squeeze that in too while living across time zones and defying the odds? I wanted to complete our family. And for me, that meant another round of *in vitro* fertility treatments (IVF) which was hell. I had lived that nightmare trying to get pregnant with Gabriel, but I'd gladly pay the price again.

I was invincible.

I also knew my body was breaking down. Something was going on. It finally hit me. Mentally, I had a weak moment and I knew what I had to do. I had to leave my job. My health forced my hand. Through tears, I told my bosses at Fox in Austin that

I'd be leaving. *That. Was. Hard.* I felt I was trading one huge, treasured chapter of my life for others that now seemed more important. The next few years would bring plenty of challenges, for sure. But I never doubted one minute that I had what it takes to conquer them. *Remember. . . I was invincible.*

I never doubted I could handle the adversity that came my way because that's what I've *always* done! And I have plenty of practice. I'm an over-comer.

My sister and I were raised in Atlanta by a Cuban immigrant father and a first-generation Italian mother, neither of whom got a college education. Our family didn't have wealth or connections. We lived modestly. On the rare occasions we dined out, we knew to order the least expensive meal on the menu and have water to drink, to make sure we didn't overspend. But we were rich in so much love, and in experience thanks to my dad's career as an airline flight dispatcher. His job allowed us to see the world for free and experience life in its far corners. I learned at a young age that making memories trumped material items any day—you can take them with you forever. Travel was eye-opening. It softened my heart, but it also fueled my drive for success and my dream to share stories with the world.

Though I had big dreams as a child, I couldn't see a way to get where I was going. Our parents didn't teach us to take risks, maybe since they'd both suffered more than their share of losses. My father, in fact, came from a family with status, money, chauffeurs, chefs, and every comfort you could imagine. All that was lost when he fled communist Cuba in 1959, ending up on the streets of New York City with not a penny to his name.

Instead, they taught us to work hard for what we wanted. Not that we had a choice—it was the only option. My strong-willed

Italian mother was driven and determined to make sure we had a better life than she had growing up.

Through that loss, my Papi always made sure we understood that life is *not* about the material things you own, or your status, but about who you are as a human being. Your drive and your character matter. No matter what challenge our family faced, Papi would always remind us, "But you have your life, health and you have your freedom, right?" He wove that message into his everyday parenting: "You can lose it *all* in an instant." I never imagined I would one day come to understand that message firsthand.

From early on, most of the opportunities I had, I made happen on my own. Playing competitive sports fueled my drive. I set goals, laid out an aggressive timeline, then followed my strategy. And when events didn't go my way, I always looked for how to turn a negative into a positive. Naysayers were just *white noise* to me.

To be sure, I did not naturally have all the ingredients to be a poised, well-spoken, confident news anchor. For starters, I grew up with a lisp. That is, I "talked funny," according to kids in my elementary school and at the bus stop. I attended speech therapy for years, but it didn't stop classmates from picking on me. The teasing and bullying left me in tears daily. Even tougher, my dream was to be a journalist and an on-air communicator. It fueled me to work harder and prove all the bullies wrong. Instead of giving in to frustration and letting a lisp come between me and my dreams, I determined to "fix" my speech issue. I devised a plan and charged ahead with it like a bull, even though success took years. With that part of the hurdle behind me, I became eager to help others overcome their *own* obstacles.

I planned everything down to a tee and then followed my strategic plan. Eventually, "Want it. Work for it. Make it happen." became the motto I lived by. If a door didn't open for me, I found a way to kick it down. And I fed off success—while I was achieving one goal, I'd be laying the groundwork for the next.

Like my older sister, Lisa, I worked my way through college taking a variety of jobs. At age nineteen, I landed a yearlong paid internship with IBM, first in Atlanta, then on to New York to work in tech support. But I wasn't making the cut, and I think management realized I was a poor match for that assignment. Yes, I knew a social butterfly like me might not make a good techie, but I thought that, for $15 an hour and college credit, I could teach myself! The day they called me in to fire me, I was so confident that at the end of the meeting I still didn't realize I was being let go.

My boss said, "I don't think you will be coming back next semester."

I said, "Great, when will you know?"

He responded, "I know. You really aren't a good fit here in tech support, but we do have to make you an offer to go to a different division to finish up your credits and commitments as a paid intern."

I replied, "Great. I want to go to SPAIN." I thought he was going to spit out his drink. "Yep, Spain."

Two weeks later, I was packing my bags for a six-month paid position at IBM in Madrid doing what I love: TALKING. They sent me to teach executives how to use their software programs and networks.

As it happens, when my job in Spain was over, I was eligible for unemployment benefits back in the U.S. Perfect! But I wasn't going to sit on my ass and watch the money roll in, I was going to use it to pay myself a salary so I could accept the *unpaid* internship of my dreams . . . at CNN and CNN en Español in Atlanta. I'd already lined it up.

I had to be closer to home because my parents were getting divorced and money was tight. I moved in with my mom to help her with the bills, enrolled in night courses eighty miles away, and fulfilled my CNN internship on the overnight shift, from 11 PM to 7 AM.

I loved being in the newsroom. But I knew I didn't want to roll the prompter forever or keep writing stories for other reporters to read on the air. If I was going to write stories, I wanted full credit for my hard work. I also noticed that many of the anchors showed up at the last minute, often unprepared, and they didn't have backup, (i.e., extra suits, clothes for various breaking stories). I felt they got complacent in their jobs. Burnout, perhaps from the long hours. So, I hatched a master scheme to achieve my goals and get to work.

First, I started buying pizza for the production staff, so they could eat their dinner while they helped me. Then, when the news anchors took a break, I hopped on the set and ran through a newscast just like it was the real deal. Oh, I also made friends with makeup artists who worked their magic and talent so I could look TV ready. I kept a suit in my locker. After CNN put me on the payroll, I got colleagues to help me make resume tapes that I would bring up to the network president's office to show off my work. Each time, Bob Furnad would shake his head and say, "Honey, you are going to have to start in Beaumont. You don't start an on-air job at a network like CNN."

I would kindly smile and say, "I don't know where Beaumont is, but my parents are in the midst of a divorce and I can't leave my mom, so my dreams are going to have to come true right here. Trust me. One day you will need me."

It took two years of buying pizza and begging friends to roll the video, but it finally happened. All my hard work was about to pay off, and I was *prepared*.

An anchor for the Headline News evening shift was stuck in traffic and couldn't get to the studio in time. The CNN president came up to me and said, "Kid, go get your suit. You are about to get your big break."

I grinned and answered with pride, "I knew you would need me!"

That day I went from rolling prompter to announcing, "Good evening from the CNN Center in Atlanta, I'm Lori Hernandez." On camera from 7 to 11 PM. I smiled through the good, the bad, and the ugly stories, but I kicked ass the entire four-hour shift. When I finished, Mr. Furnad came up to me and said, "Great job! We need to get you some official training and some coaching, but you are on your way. Let's meet two times a week for on-air training."

Woo-hoo!!! At the time I was still juggling a college class schedule, but there was no way I was going to miss this opportunity. I got to the studio very early for training on the set when the real anchors had breaks. We practiced breaking-news scenarios. I struggled and screwed up for a while, but then it clicked.

Soon I was meeting with a voice coach to help me get rid of my accent and an image coach to help me look perfect for TV—no double-breasted suits (they make you look bigger), only

V-necks (they make your neck look longer), thin out your eyebrows, cut your hair, throw some fake eyelashes on to open your eyes more—I was like a new person in the making. Next thing I knew, I was sitting around the table with executives pouring over my presentation, delivery style, and "look." Mr. Furnad had them watching tapes of my practice sessions and critiquing *every single thing* I did. It was wild and intimidating. But I knew if I wanted to make it at CNN, I'd better have thick skin and listen to every word they said.

I eagerly agreed to all the changes—even their suggestion that I keep my name as "Lori." I wanted the world to know me as "Loriana Hernández," adding an accent, but they thought that was too much for viewers to handle (a clear sign of the times and lack of diversity then). These days that would never fly, but I was young and wanted to soar in my career. You could call me anything, just let me be on the air as an anchor and reporter. Those weren't the times you could stand up for diversity and inclusion and actually get somewhere. My strategy was to just get my career launched and then switch to Loriana. That's exactly what I ended up doing.

Before long I was juggling two jobs—permanent fill-in anchor and production assistant, where I would roll prompter and transcribe interviews for reporters. I would go in to work, do the fonts for a show (the supertitles identifying people on screen), run up to makeup, and then get on the set wherever an anchor was needed—either at Headline News, the Airport Network or the CNN Newsroom kids' show.

I'd started my unpaid internship at age twenty. Within three months I was officially on staff, and in two years I was anchoring and reporting the news. And not in Beaumont!

I prepared for everything.

I thrived off of game plans.

Nothing got in my way as I reached for my dreams. Nothing. I overcame long odds to build a successful television career at CNN headquarters, followed by stints at local stations around California and Texas. I created an on-air "brand" by reporting diet, fitness, and medical issues, coaching viewers to make healthier choices. Along the way I met and married a loving, supportive partner who shared my passions—even though our jobs kept us in distant cities. We produced a healthy, beautiful son—even after doctors told us I couldn't conceive.

I made it my habit to defy the odds.

CHAPTER 3

The Fall

The plan was for us to move out of the Austin house in January. Cesar would drive my car to Washington, and Gabriel and I would stay behind for a couple of days at the home of a friend who was traveling. That way I could finish fertility treatments, and as soon as the embryo transplant was done, my boy and I could hop on a plane.

Everything was in place, just like I had always arranged things. The only way I could justify leaving Austin with my head up was making it not about my health and exhaustion but rather a need to leave because of a baby on the way. After all, I was the health and fitness reporter. The clean-eating, green-drinking yoga enthusiast. I couldn't help others transform their lives and let mine publicly fall apart. I had an image to uphold, right?

I continued giving myself fertility injections in the stomach. As the IVF transfer approached, I wore estrogen patches to boost my hormone levels. And we finally had a due date for the baby—October 11, 2014. I'd be a mom again, and our family of four was going to be glorious! I tried to convince myself that if I had another baby, my health would quickly fall back into place.

At last, it was moving day. Cesar flew in to help and to collect the car and our dog, Isabella. My dad and my stepmom, Jane, arrived to ride back with her across the country.

But as the movers were packing the house, Gabriel didn't feel well. I took him to a nearby urgent care center. Then when we got home, I didn't feel well and began to throw up. It had to be the flu, my nerves, the hormones, or the denial as to why I was leaving a high-profile successful career. In my heart, I didn't want to leave (my health forced my hand). Cesar hated to leave me that way, but I told him to get on the road and I kissed him goodbye.

I buckled Gabriel into the backseat of my rental car and locked the house behind me for the last time. Now shaking and violently vomiting as I drove, I finally made it to "my friend Lorraine's house," where we would stay. Gabriel cried the whole way. I was covered in vomit. But I knew Lorraine had two friends house-sitting and I figured they could help me. I pulled into her driveway, leaving Gabriel in the car, and ran to the door, where I screamed and collapsed. "Get my son, get my son," I pleaded. "Just take care of him for me." They brought me inside and laid me down on Lorraine's bed. I was violently ill. *Violently!!!* I couldn't function.

Even then—*even then!* —I was determined to push through with the plan. Crying, I called my fertility specialist and told him, "I'm throwing up, but I'll be at your office tomorrow, ready for my lab work and ready to have this baby."

But Dr. Shar Kavoussi, who had already made my dream to be a mom come true with Gabriel less than two years ago, wanted one more blood test just to show I was 100 percent healthy. He told me a successful transfer would depend on me being healthy. But that's not what the test found.

A couple days later Dr. Kavoussi called and asked if he could come see me to discuss something. I immediately got upset and a bit angry. Had he lost or damaged our only remaining embryos? (By the way, even to this day, we are still paying to store those embryos. I can't seem to find closure to let go.) Although he and I had a great doctor-patient relationship, even a friendship, I was furious as I waited for him to show up at Lorraine's house.

When I opened the door, his face was drawn and his body was trembling. I knew something was terribly wrong. What would I say to him if in fact he *had* lost our precious embryos? How could I politely vent my rage? He did, after all, give me my angel, Gabriel. Dr. Kavoussi came inside, sat down and held my hand. Tears rolled down his face as he said, "You can't have a second baby. You have cancer. Leukemia."

I looked at Gabriel on my lap and the room started to spin. I sobbed and screamed, telling him he was crazy. The results *couldn't* be right. After all, his field was fertility, not oncology. And I knew a thing or two about cancer since for years I'd been coaching all my viewers about how to avoid it—at well and keep in shape *like I did.*

I insisted we redo the test. The very next day I drove like a lunatic back to the lab to have more blood drawn. Carrying Gabriel in my arms, I walked in and asked to see the phlebotomist. "Weren't you just here?" she asked. "We already drew this lab."

"Draw it again," I trembled and demanded, through tears. "You guys messed up."

23

Once again, Dr. Kavoussi called me to report. "I'm so sorry but the test is right. My heart aches for you, but you have cancer. You need help."

I got connected to Austin's top oncologist. That doctor read the two lab reports and disputed the cancer diagnosis. Yes, disputed them!

I knew it! I knew it all along!

He looked me in the eyes. "You will have this baby," he promised. "You are healthy but you're run down. Just start saying 'no' to things and get more rest."

Still, to appease Dr. Kavoussi, he scheduled a bone-marrow biopsy for later in the week. "Go out and enjoy the night," the oncologist told me.

I did!

That night, I celebrated with my friends and toasted with champagne over such a mix up! What a night. Whew. What a scare!

I was in such denial.

The day of my biopsy, another friend (Lisa Rice, my clean-eating plant-based chef) watched Gabriel. I confidently strutted into the hospital, even laughing with the staff. Like everything else in my life, I was going to have my dreams come true because of hard work and determination. IVF had been tough, but I knew I was tougher.

> Remember, I was invincible, much like many are thinking when it comes to COVID-19 and other illnesses.

This was just an extra challenge.

Friday evening, the oncologist was going to phone with the pathology report from the biopsy. My girlfriend Tracy insisted on hanging out with me at Lorraine's until he called. I thought that was silly, since all the doctor was going to do was tell me I was fine—while her kids and husband were home waiting for dinner.

Around 8 PM the phone rang. The oncologist's voice cracked as he stuttered, talking round and round about I can't remember what. I do remember finally telling him, "Get to the point! What are the damn results?"

The doctor stuttered again. "You . . . You . . . you have cancer. Leukemia. Call my office Monday afternoon to discuss."

That was it.

I handed the phone to Tracy, ran and grabbed my baby, and screamed at the top of my lungs.

What the hell was happening to me? Was I going to die? What was "leukemia"? I had no idea, even though I vaguely recalled doing several on-air fundraisers for the cause countless times in my career. I realized then that it never really clicked. It never does until it actually hits home, right? I imagined I could just go "fix" my cancer with some chemotherapy or whatever it took—like I'd fixed all my problems my whole life. I had spoken at countless "Leukemia & Lymphoma Society" events. I even trained for "Team in Training"—an LLS-developed running program to run races and raise money for blood cancers—yet I didn't remember what a blood cancer was. When it was finally *my* story, it was like I had never heard the word. I didn't know there were so many kinds, or that the stakes were so high.

That's often how it works, right? We never truly understand a cause until we are personally affected. I realized at that moment I never really understood what I was raising money for except to make a difference.

I froze and stared into space. Finally, I called Cesar, who had just arrived at the house in Virginia where the movers were unpacking our things. I put the phone on speaker and shrieked at the top of my lungs, "I have cancerrrrrrrrrrrr!!!" My husband had no clue what I was saying. Tracy took the phone from me and told him, "Get on a plane, Loriana has cancer!" In the background, I was screaming like a lunatic.

After the call, Cesar—who is an expert in crisis management in the broadcast industry and never shows his emotions—sat on the bare wooden floor and wept. Why were we being punished? He called his best friend, Joe, and broke down telling him the news.

As the movers hurriedly stacked the remaining boxes inside the doorway, Cesar called the Leukemia & Lymphoma Society, hoping for direction. Tracy had thought to write down the doctor's scary words: "acute myeloid leukemia." AML. Then he headed to the airport.

Back in Texas, I didn't know what to do. So many years of my television career I'd spent advocating as a news anchor and reporter, and suddenly *I* became the damn story. I went from telling everyone's story to becoming the story. I never in a million years thought that would happen through cancer. It was embarrassing. I realized I'd need to put my head before my heart and focus just like I had done countless times covering other tragic stories that drove me to tears. I could only be helpful if I asked the tough questions and was willing to share the answers. So, I went into reporter mode.

Saturday was a big blur.

My first order of business was making sure I would *never* have to see that oncologist again—not Monday afternoon, not *ever*. There was NO WAY I was going to sit around and wait to get a game plan when my life was at stake.

I did what I knew as a journalist: I researched my subject, then hit social media to put the word out about my diagnosis. I begged my followers for help and any leads to a great oncologist. My station even went on the air with my diagnosis. *This was my breaking news.*

Immediately, my cell phone began to ding with texts and ring with calls, and it didn't stop. People I knew—and even viewers I didn't—overwhelmed me with so many cancer stories. Cancers I didn't even have. Not leukemia, not even blood cancer stories. Cancers that required totally different treatments than acute myeloid leukemia (AML).

They told upbeat stories. "You will be fine. My aunt survived x-y-z cancer after three weeks of treatment." Or stories of loss. "I understand your stress, my dad died of leukemia."

Some asked, "How does the fitness reporter, queen of what not to eat, and host of the 'Clean Eating' health segment get leukemia?"

What?

But other friends in the media also started digging for answers. I was amazed how many connections we all had; friends of friends of friends. Who knew that someone's cousin's ex-boyfriend had a stepfather who's chief of oncology in I-Forget-Where? It was humbling.

To free me up to do research, I made Cesar the point person for all the incoming calls. And through the madness and confusion, the sky opened with people offering leads to incredible doctors and other resources.

At that moment, I realized how connected I was. This was a different kind of privilege. Yet, while I accepted every bit of help, connections made and doors opened for me, I felt some guilt for those who didn't have the same privilege. I looked at Cesar and said, "How do other patients get the help they need if they aren't connected?"

I forged ahead. My son needed me. I wasn't going to turn down the high-end world-renowned doctors, but it was that day that the term "health disparities" finally hit home to me. It wasn't from all the medical reports I did on health disparities. It was from living it and being blessed to be on the other side of it.

I was about to get better care and get it immediately.

We learned that acute myeloid leukemia has no recognized cure, and that at the time, the treatment for AML had not changed in forty years. The *only* option for me would be repeated rounds of very toxic chemo dripped into my veins.

Then, thanks to social media, the Leukemia & Lymphoma Society and all that outpouring of support, I found the most incredible doctor, Dr. Mark Levis of Johns Hopkins University, at the Sidney Kimmel Cancer Center. My HERO. In fact, so many people called Dr. Levis on my behalf that he called me that Sunday morning at 5 AM. "We have a bed waiting for you," he said. "You don't have time to wait. Get on a plane to Baltimore now."

And then: "Say goodbye to your son. Sign over guardianship, and give him to your mom to care for."

It was really happening. I scrambled to pack a few clothes while Cesar booked my flight. He rushed us to the airport.

We got a speeding ticket on the way. Who gives a ticket to a man crying that his wife has cancer?

I brought Gabriel with me to the gate while Cesar got rid of the rental car. My best friend, Craig, stayed with us. I was on the phone giving interviews to other media outlets about my story while I held Gabriel, who was clinging and sobbing. After the very last call to board the flight, I looked at Gabriel in his eyes and said, "Baby, please know that Mami will *always* love you. Know I gave it my all. Know I will do anything for you. Please remember me, my love."

I loosened the grip of his little arms around my neck and handed him to Craig, who would take him to Cesar. As I boarded the plane, Gabriel's cries of "Mami, Mami!" echoed down the jetway. Those words play over and over and over in my head. The PTSD from that moment will never go away. The hole in my heart from that moment will stay forever.

At that moment, I didn't know if I would ever see my child again.

I feared that if cancer didn't kill me, I might die of a broken heart.

But I knew I needed to go. It was my only option. If I wanted any chance at being able to watch him grow up, this was it.

The sting of that day was worse than any drip of chemo that would flow through my veins.

Cesar would fly with Gabriel to Atlanta, literally handing him over to my sister at the baggage claim before getting back on a plane to Baltimore. Lisa would deliver our toddler to my seventy-year-old mother to keep—while I underwent treatment and Cesar somehow kept functioning at his new, senior leadership job in Maryland. Dad and Jane took the dog.

The household we'd been pulling back together was shattered into parts.

Flying alone across the country, I stared numbly out the window for what felt like the longest trip of my life. I was terrified, and for once I had nothing to say. Cesar's friend Joe and his amazing wife Tracey were the only two people I knew in the D.C. metro area. Tracey greeted me at the BWI terminal outside Baltimore and let me cry in her arms. It was such a relief to have her there to witness the start of an ordeal I couldn't quite believe was happening. She was a busy makeup artist for the Fox Network, with political and other celebrity clients, so I didn't want to be a burden on her time. But I needed her to share my fears with, thousands of miles away from my familiar support system. Tracey drove us to Johns Hopkins, where they were waiting to admit me, and she stayed by my side as long as she could.

Eventually, Cesar arrived, straight from the airport. He walked in with his head down, looking defeated. Hours before, he'd handed over our son in Atlanta. I felt horrible, trying to imagine the burden my husband was carrying. What had I done?

The hospital staff had taken my insurance information. Then they wanted to know if I had an advance medical directive--or a will. *Well, no, I never thought . . .*

We never think it will be us. COVID-19 should be your reminder that it can be you. Do you have your will or advanced directive ready?

That very night they put a catheter called a Hickman in my chest. The tubing allows the nurses to hook up a bag of chemo drugs directly to that port. From there the chemo flows straight into your heart, to be pumped out to the rest of your body.

The walls spun around and I saw that my bed was surrounded by a team of rounding doctors, nurses, researchers analyzing my case—some of medicine's best in the world. But I was still in denial.

They re-tested my blood to confirm that what I had was, in fact, leukemia. Then they confirmed it was AML. The most difficult form of the disease to treat. The most fatal of them all. The odds were against me.

A million hormone patches still plastered my stomach, in preparation for the IVF embryo transfer. There was no way in hell I would let them peel those off. Just the day before—even after being told I had cancer—I had gone ahead with the final progesterone shot because I was so sure this was all a damn mistake. I was going to have my baby.

Now there was a team of Johns Hopkins doctors, nurses, and a social worker surrounding my bed. About eight of them. They told me again what I refused to believe, "You have leukemia, you might die. You cannot have a baby."

Bullshit. I kicked and screamed. I couldn't handle it. I cried and asked if they could harvest more of my eggs, to fertilize and implant after the chemo worked. To do that, they would need to delay my cancer treatment by fourteen days. They told me I didn't have fourteen days to wait because my life was in jeopardy. I was so sick. Violently ill. The symptoms, similar to COVID-19 in many ways. I needed chemo NOW. But I so badly wanted Gabriel to have a sibling and keep my dreams alive. I begged to see a specialist, refusing to believe that it wasn't possible. Surely, I was invincible. The doctors may as well have been talking to a wall.

I asked Cesar to meet with them, and he looked at me like I'd lost my mind. In fact, at that point the team didn't think I was mentally "fit" to make a decision to delay treatment. I wasn't. Cesar made the choice for me, that we would not wait, but would move forward with my potentially life-saving but body-damaging chemo.

I was so pissed.

I was so devastated. There was no shared decision making. It was decision made. Without me. Maybe I'm alive because my doctor and husband made that decision for me. We will never know.

To this day I can barely talk about that huge loss. The pain in my heart has never healed, and October 11th — our baby's due date — has never been the same.

***

I would be staying at Johns Hopkins. I had cancer. I wasn't going to have another baby. I barely slept that night, though I was exhausted.

Early the next morning Dr. Levis came to explain the treatment plan and prognosis to me and Cesar. He had reviewed my test results and case history with the other doctors and specialists at the Sidney Kimmel Comprehensive Cancer Center.

"We will need you for the next year," he said.

I couldn't believe the words that came out of his mouth "... *the next year.*" Not a few days, or a couple of weeks, as I imagined. *What?*

Suddenly, "*I am invincible*" didn't have the same ring.

I wasn't.

I became the story.

And my discovery and breaking news were about to be the biggest story of my career.

CHAPTER 4

Prehabilitation, Discovery, and Hospital Voids

My M.O. my entire life has been to be prepared and set myself up for success. It was about to prove true in ways I never imagined. It's where I was forced into an emotional growth and discovery like many are going through now with COVID. It's where I turned my thoughts of shame as a then-sick on-air "transformational health coach" into one of inspiration, as I uncovered and discovered the 3Ps to surviving illness.

I call it: PREPARE—PRESENT—PREVAIL ®

Before I dive into what the 3Ps stand for and how I discovered them years ago during my leukemia battle, let me say this about COVID-19.

Preparation matters for everyone—both the healthcare system and the patient. If we want to drive patient outcomes, the patient must meet the medicine halfway and the healthcare system must meet us (the patient) halfway. The more prepared the healthcare system is with necessary equipment like respirators and personal protection equipment like gloves and masks, the more lives are saved. The more prepared the medical teams are to treat the whole patient, the better the outcomes. While my incredible world-renowned oncologist saved my life, the system itself in some ways failed me by not giving me the tools I needed for success in order to emotionally cope and physically navigate survivorship.

On the flip side, the better prepared a patient is, the better he or she can physically fight and better position himself/herself to win.

Preparedness on both sides is crucial for success.

But thanks to my yearlong leukemia battle, I was a veteran of this war (COVID) long before it started. I got a five-year jumpstart on what the world learned in 2020: preparedness matters. I got a jumpstart on the germ warfare, wearing N95 masks daily, isolation, managing loneliness, droplet precautions, what it was truly like to be on death's door, and how devastating it was to lose friends one-by-one while I stayed standing. The PTSD never eases up.

Yes, Leukemia was MY COVID-19. . . my wake-up call.
Leukemia is a cancer of blood cells and the bone marrow that produces them; that means it was circulating everywhere in my body. There's no cure for my type—Acute Myeloid Leukemia (AML)—which rapidly corrupts the new white blood cells that normally fight off infections. For my AML, Dr. Levis explained, he had basically two roads to choose from. LLS has launched a BEAT AML Master Trial to help with treatment breakthroughs, and some have been made since I was diagnosed in 2014, but there's more work to be done.

The most effective and aggressive approach would be a bone marrow transplant to replace the cancerous cells, after a few weeks of toxic chemotherapy to kill them off. But transplants are high risk. They don't always "take," and deadly infections are common when your immune system is destroyed. The medical team knew I had a young child at home who needed his mom.

Dr. Levis said the safer approach would be HIDAC, which stands for high intensity doses of a chemotherapy drug called ARA-C. The idea was to kill my white blood cells through four or five cycles of intravenous chemo. Every time my white blood cell count got knocked down to zero, the new cells that grew back should be cancer free according to Dr. Levis. They'd check my bone marrow with excruciating bone marrow biopsies two weeks later to confirm the results. But each round (which start to finish can take twenty-five to forty-five days, and after a few rounds when your body is tired it can eventually take about eighty days) gets harder and takes longer, since the toxic drug compounds itself and builds up and your resistance breaks down. It could be ten or twelve months altogether (not days . . . months!) in isolation on the cancer ward, because everyday germs can quickly kill a person who has no immune resistance. Everyday germs like the ones small children collect (Dr. Levis described kids as "Petri dishes"). Small children like my son, Gabriel.

And if the HIDAC chemo didn't work, he warned, I might still need a bone marrow transplant, if my body could handle it.

My prognosis for surviving the whole treatment cycle and living another five years, Dr. Levis told me, was 25 percent. Twenty-five percent! I can do math. That meant 75 percent I'd be dead before Gabriel turned seven.

I was in shock. But what choice did I have? Fine, I thought, let me sign on the dotted line and let's get this done! I just wanted to hold my baby boy. To me, the best plan was the one that would let me be Gabriel's mom again, ASAP.

Dr. Levis nodded. "Put your armor on," he said. "Keep moving and stay focused and stay fit, so we can try to get you home to your son." They don't talk in black and white and guarantees; doctors on the cancer unit talk in grays, which include "we will try," "we will do our best," and "our goal is." It drove me CRAZY.

TAKEAWAY

Learn how to ArmorUp for LIFE®.

I had no idea what was in store for me.

It was time to start Round 1 of the HIDAC therapy that loomed ahead of me. The nurses gave me a calendar for my wall detailing the schedule for that phase of treatment. On the calendar it noted the days I would get doses of IV chemo, and the days I would rest. It gave numbers for what my blood counts should be at different points, with spaces to write in the actual levels along the way. Oh, and around Day 14 my hair would fall out, the calendar predicted. Ha! Not mine, I was sure.

Sadly, nowhere on the calendar did it say when I would get to see Gabriel again. Nowhere did I get emotional help to cope with the separation. I had to ask to see the psychologist, and when she stopped by it was a ten-minute visit. Brilliant as she might be, she was unprepared and far from helpful. She was a waste of my time. She didn't know my cancer well and I found myself explaining to her why I couldn't see my son. The psy-cho-oncology part of this process was non-existent. Apparently, the timing would depend on my response to the toxic chemo, how long it took to kill my cancerous cells, and then the time it took to build me back up to a safe place.

The goal is for chemo to wipe out the cancerous blood cells. But there's no way to keep healthy cells from getting damaged, too. So, the drugs wipe out all your blood cells—good, bad and ugly. This is why precision medicine and advancements matter. Once your "counts" drop to zero, you wait for your body to start slowly regenerating replacement cells. You build up your resistance to a target level. When you're strong enough, you get to do it all over again with the next round of chemo. Great.

For some people, the chemo is deadlier than the cancer—and their blood cells never start producing again. It's like trying to rev a new engine that just won't start. That's why doctors carefully tailor the chemo dosage for each patient, then adjust it constantly. The more your body can handle, the more aggres-sively they can treat you and the bigger the dose you might get. It's the opposite if they have to tiptoe around other illnesses you showed up with—like diabetes, heart disease, or high blood pressure. The more fit you are, the better you can fight. But only later would I fully understand that.

Of course, they warn you that the chemo has side effects such as diarrhea, excruciating pain, swelling, weight changes, mood changes, nausea, and impaired overall brain function. It's spelled out in tiny print—and you sign paperwork that says you are aware of that. Not to mention I didn't look like myself. But if you are like me, at that point you don't really give a shit. What else can you do, so why bother reading? It's either die now or suffer later, so "Hurry up and let's get this shit going" was my attitude. I wanted to get in, get out, and start my second chance, living a completely different way than I did before. That didn't mean a new diet or workout plan. I ate clean and worked out. That meant getting rid of the stress in my life, meditating more, and limiting the toxicity in my life.

One more step: They also bring you a cognitive questionnaire to fill out ("What year is it? What's your name?" and other basic facts) and assign you something to draw. This is to test your mental capacity *before* you get chemo, then you do it again *after* every round. I laughed each time I drew the picture or answered the questions. This meant nothing to me. I mean, I am dying and I'm really going to say, "Well hmmm, I don't like this side effect, so yeah, I'll skip my treatment today." Only later did I realize how many ways I'd always taken my mind for granted. You always think the damage won't happen to you, until you live and suffer through each and every side effect both short and long-term. Now, I know the price I paid.

TAKEAWAY

Additional side effects from chemo:

- Hair loss
- Easy bruising and bleeding
- Infection
- Anemia (low red blood cell counts)
- Appetite and weight changes

- Constipation
- Mouth, tongue, and throat problems, such as sores and pain with swallowing
- Peripheral neuropathy or other nerve problems, i.e., numbness, tingling, and pain
- Skin and nail changes, such as dry skin and color change
- Urine and bladder changes and kidney problems
- "Chemo brain," which can affect concentration and focus
- Changes in sexual function

LONG-TERM SIDE EFFECTS:

Once you survive, there are these side effects to look for. I call them collateral damage. It depends on what chemo and dosages you have, but for me, I had all of these and then some.

Not all chemotherapy medicines have the same late effects. A lot depends on the kind of medicines used. The dosage and whether chemotherapy was done with another type of treatment are also important. NOTE: PREVIOUS SENTENCES ARE REDUNDANT TO PREVIOUS PARAGRAPH Long-term side effects include:

- Fatigue
- Difficulty with focused thinking (sometimes called "chemo brain) IF YOU ARE DEFINING IT, YOU NEED TO DEFINE IT THE FIRST TIME YOU USE IT
- Early menopause
- Heart problems
- Reduced lung capacity
- Kidney and urinary problems
- Nerve problems such as numbness and tingling
- Bone and joint problems

- Muscle weakness
- Secondary cancers

Let's not even think about what radiation does to the body, and for blood cancers, it isn't just targeted to one specific area—it is FULL-BODY radiation. The cancer is running through your blood. Again, another reason I am grateful that there are new treatments being fast-tracked that are less toxic:

- Cataracts
- Dry mouth
- Problems with thyroid or adrenal glands
- Infertility
- Slowed or halted bone growth in children
- Decreased range of motion in the treated area
- Skin sensitivity to sun exposure
- Problems with memory or ability to learn
- Cancers

A pair of nurses came in to start the first IV drip of liquid ARA-C into my chest. They were fully masked and covered up in yellow isolation gowns personal protection equipment (PPE) to protect them from the toxic drugs in the bag, which was double-wrapped in gauze. One read out my ID number from the chart—*8556XXXX*—and the second repeated it aloud from the label on the bag—*8556XXXX*—to confirm that the medicine was going to the correct patient. Like a military check. The delivery would take twelve hours.

Cesar had gone to work that morning in Bethesda, Maryland, at NBC Sports putting in his usual long, high-pressure day. Then late in the evening he drove back to the hospital in Baltimore to sleep in yellow isolation gear on the pull-out couch in my room. No hand holding. No hugging. No human touch. My husband would do this every night for most of a year, going home to Virginia only to get clean clothes once a week. Cesar was my rock, but inside I knew my cancer was nearly killing him inside.

Those first few days of chemo I didn't yet feel the physical effects. So, when I wasn't getting a chemo drip, I strutted around the cancer unit and walked all over the hospital like a speed racer. That is, a speed racer pushing an IV pole on rollers! For a whole year, I was permanently tethered to that IV, like a leash. It's how I received dozens of medicines and hydration fluids, and how they took three-times-a-day blood draws. It went everywhere with me.

"Keep moving," Dr. Levis had urged me. One day in bed, he explained, will set you back four days in muscle strength—and four days in bed can erase a whole month of strength. Wow, this was powerful. *This is a story.* I see everything as content for stories to share and stories to tell. Why didn't I do a story on this in my twenty-plus years on television?

He explained, "You cannot afford not to move, because eventually, you will lose the will to get back up and fight." Lying down too long allows fluid to build up in your lungs, which risks pneumonia—a common cause of death for patients who stay bedridden. Much like we hear about with COVID-19 patients, pneumonia can take you before the actual illness does. "It happens often here," my oncologist said.

I took his message to heart. I was terrified to lie down. No way was I going to let pneumonia take me before the cancer could. I walked and walked and walked, counting seventy-two laps around the fifth floor to equal one mile! It helped me cope and feel some sense of control.

Each afternoon I would pull myself together, put on a smile, and call my mom in Atlanta for a video chat with Gabriel. She'd put him on her phone, and there—right there!—would be his confused little face. I'd try not to let him see me fighting back tears, or how my heart was breaking to be so far away. I would sometimes turn my phone away for a moment to sob and then move it back and fake a smile and a happy pitched voice. Only a few weeks before, I was breastfeeding him. After every call, there was plenty of time to cry.

Then all at once, the treatment hit me like a ton of bricks. Like the most horrendous, most violent flu—like we hear about with COVID patients, except this was every single day. It never let up. For a year, I was so weak. I spent all day on my hands and knees crawling between bed and the bathroom, either puking or with diarrhea. Buckets of it. The techs begged me, "Ma'am, there are so many germs on the floor! Please let us get someone to help you, to carry you." I thought for sure death was near. But as I cried and crawled, I heard flashbacks of my son's voice on the video link, asking, "Mami, how many more sleeps?" I could not give up. The PTSD was just getting started. A disorder that would cripple me for years after I survived.

Things weren't going well down in Atlanta. One day, barely into my second week at Johns Hopkins, I was hooked up to an IV chemo drip. My phone rang, and the hysterical person calling was my seventy-year-old mother. "I can't do this alone; you have to get me help!" she yelled. "Gabriel is in pieces without you. He needs to see you. And I'm having a mental breakdown! I'm an exhausted wreck and I can't stand watching him suffer."

My mom hadn't been in charge of a toddler for forty years, let alone one who was suddenly facing multiple traumas—including a strange house and separation from his parents. And she wasn't prepared for it. Who could be?

But I was furious. I screamed back that I didn't want to hear about it even if the world was ending—I was busy trying to save my own life! She'd have to solve this herself. Or at least make me think everything was fine, because the pain of being away from my child was sucking the life out of me. "Handle it! Just handle it!" I said. "I have chemo running through my veins. Tell me it's all perfect down there; that's what I need to know."

Of course, as soon as we hung up, I went online to try to find child care options near her house. In Georgia. I had no idea how we would pay for that. I was so frightened; everything was falling apart. But I knew right then I couldn't die, I just couldn't die.

"Stay focused," Dr. Levis had said. And how was I supposed to do that?

The side effects got worse. I got shingles on my ass, and the nerve pain was unreal. Every inch of my body ached—including my bones (typical for leukemia). I couldn't keep a thing down, and I developed mucositis—ulcers in my digestive tract and blisters in my mouth. That meant I couldn't swallow, so I had to take fluids and nutrition intravenously. I needed Cesar to bathe me, and to help feed me those times I was able to take in soft food.

But I'd always pick myself up and keep walking, or at least shuffling, if that's what I could manage. And not just a few laps around the hallways like they suggested, but two miles—sometimes four or five by the end of the day. I had a son waiting for me and I was not going down for good.

I kept wondering to myself: If I was in good enough shape to have finished triathlons and half-marathons, and I'm already struggling to tolerate this cancer treatment, how the hell does anyone who shows up not fit survive this?

Like a good reporter, I went looking for answers. Uncertainty and a broken heart would kill me, I was certain, even if the cancer didn't.

On Day 14 my hair fell out, just like they said it would. Big chunks of beautiful, dark hair. The hair I spent years learning to style for the TV cameras, the hair Gabriel once clung to when he nursed.

But I missed the chance for the hospital salon to shave it. A snow storm arrived and I needed my head shaved. That meant Cesar driving to Target in the storm to return with clippers to start on what would be many losses in my life and my identity. That night, as tears rolled down my face, Cesar tenderly shaved my head, because I'd refused the hospital's offer to do so ahead of time. I cried and cried. Another loss. They were piling up.

Looking at my strange bald head in the mirror, I was scared what Gabriel would think the next time he saw me on a video chat. Was I supposed to wear a hat? And tell him what? Who do you even ask about such a thing?

Thank God for the Nurses

The nurses at Johns Hopkins 5B (on the leukemia unit, to be exact) and others I was blessed to work with were terrific. Since most days I had no one to keep me company, the nurses became family. They understood how tough it was on me that the many people in my life who loved and cared about me couldn't be present physically. The few people I knew in the D.C. area had demanding jobs but still did their best to visit. And I was grateful when new friends from our neighborhood took the time and trouble to drive over from Virginia. But that didn't fill twenty-four hours a day, and I was usually awake for about twenty.

The nurses picked up extra items for me at the grocery store, and secretly took my laundry home to wash with theirs. They looked out for me 24/7. I was in awe of their kindness.

Sometimes after one of my walks, I would hang out at the nurse's station just to chat—about life, my fears, their kids. I adored them. They were my heroes and my friends.

And they had their hands full taking care of patients in even worse shape than I was. They were lifting 300-pound patients. They were getting screamed at by stressed-out relatives whose mothers, fathers, brothers, or sisters were struggling to stay alive. They went nonstop, all with smiles on their faces and love in their hearts.

So, I took it upon myself to handle what I needed if they were engaged elsewhere. My total lack of patience was another contributing factor. When I hit the intercom buzzer on my bed to ask for something I needed, I was only going to hit it once. I would wait about sixty seconds, and if I didn't hear a voice over the speaker that was fine—I got my ass up and went to get it myself.

They called me a "walkie-talkie" patient. I had no time for cancer, no time for waiting and I was on a mission, with a million questions. The wheels were always turning.

The nurses laughed when I would grab my own warm blanket from the linen supply room. They would say, "Ms. Hernandez-Aldama, if you would give me just thirty seconds more, I would get it." Nope . . . no time.

Nope. No patience. If God blessed me with the strength to walk, then dammit I was going to use my feet to go solve whatever I had buzzed the nurse's station about. If it was a question or a problem, I knew where to track down the right person to ask. I was sick, so I shuffled, but it was another excuse to keep moving. They were overwhelmed—often delivering critical care to fragile patients much sicker than I was. Besides, it wasn't their job to coach me and my struggling family through a series of crises.

In fact, it seemed to be nobody's job.

I was angry, and I was terrified. When I should have been enjoying building a new nest for my reunited family, my mind was filled with worries—money, child care, the stresses on Cesar and my mother (not to mention the likelihood of dying). And I felt abandoned: deprived of the friends and community that could support me, and unseen, in some ways, by the very health care system that held my only hope for survival. There was NO emotional support. No psycho-oncology. It was yet another void in the system.

Dr. Levis could see my frustration and despair. One afternoon he stopped by my fifth-floor room in the leukemia unit, where I was hooked up for that day's seemingly endless *drip-drip-drip* of chemo.

I was feeling overwhelmed, and way past fed up. I wanted nothing more than to rip that IV out of my chest and walk out of the ward. If it weren't for the fact that my son needed me back alive, I was ready to surrender and give up. I was exhausted and running on fumes. I was on death's doorstep and almost ready to say, "take me." After all, I'd pushed myself to ridiculous lengths to keep myself healthy, and now it seemed like that wasn't worth a damn.

But that day, Dr. Levis said something that turned my world around.

What he said became the biggest story of my career. It was my breaking news!!!

"Instead of being angry about how you laid the seeds of your illness with your sleep deprivation and stress or how healthy you lived your life before you got here, be thankful that you showed up fit," he suggested. "Be grateful that you showed up prepared. One of our biggest challenges in healthcare is how patients present. We can have all the advancements in the world, but if a patient isn't fit enough to take it, it does no good."

Be grateful? Was this guy for real? I thought to myself.

"Look around you when you walk through the halls. Not everyone shows up fit enough to fight this disease," Dr. Levis continued. "You might all have the same subset of leukemia, but you can't all fight the same.

"If your heart isn't strong enough, your blood pressure isn't good enough, your weight isn't healthy enough, and we have to tiptoe around other health problems, we doctors have to drop your dose of chemo. We can't kill you trying to save you."

You only get as much medicine as you can handle, he was saying. Your dosage depends on your overall fitness . . . . Basically, how you *PRESENT.*

I was stunned. It was the most profound statement I'd heard in all my time in medical reporting. But I had questions. What about the others? The man in the next room, severely overweight, or the frail woman on an oxygen tank. Another patient had a smoker's cough, and others were clearly out of shape.

He said, "I can't tell you because of privacy rules, but you are a smart lady. When you walk the halls, take note of the chemo bags hanging from the IV stands. You will see they are all different sizes."

I looked at the bag of fluid hanging above me. It was the biggest one on the unit—by far—I knew.

Dr. Levis said, "So trust me when I say I can't promise that you will live, but I can tell you that your entire life, you *prepared* for this battle. You did everything physically right.

"You *prehabilitated*. You '*presented* well,'" he continued, using the phrase for what doctors find they have to work with when a patient shows up needing care. And that means, he says, "you have positioned yourself with the best possible chance to PREVAIL."

At that moment, the lightbulb came on for me. How we live our lives, how much exercise we do, what we fuel our bodies with, the communities we build—and our habits around stress, spirituality, and finances—will help determine how well each of us can fight when it's our turn to step into the ring.

Dr. Levis's words brought me calm, and gave me a sense of control that I deeply needed. One that people desperately need during COVID. I finally understood that I had a good start, and I was determined to *prevail*. I would get through this and survive.

Wow! I had stumbled onto the biggest news story of my career! A story that somehow, I had never covered, in all my years of transformational health, fitness, and medical reporting for viewers.

This story was way bigger than me.

I wanted to shout it from the mountaintop: Fitness is not just about getting into the skinny jeans, and it may not even successfully prevent illness. News flash—bad things can still happen to you! What matters is how well YOU prepare yourself, and the support systems you put in place.

> I thank God every single day that I showed up prepared. I was the clean-eating, green-drinking yoga enthusiast. The on-air transformational health coach. I may have laid the groundwork for my illness with my lack of sleep, but physically my body was so ready for a fight.

You must take an active role in how you "pre-habilitate" because if you don't, your body will do it for you and you won't be ready. I'm either your coach or your cautionary tale. You have the chance to be your own hero and start today. The choice is yours.

Prepare, by staying fit. Present well, and prevail. The three P's! I unofficially have a 4th P; my friends have chosen as I find myself pushing for answers and advocate for myself—Pain in the Ass. I'm alive! I'll take it.

Once again, the doctor told me, "Put your armor on, focus, and fight hard."

This time I knew what to do, and I knew it was up to me to share that discovery with the world. Then and there, from my hospital bedside, I raised the battle cry of ArmorUp for LIFE®.

Sharing that message with the world started with talking to patients right on my unit. When I didn't see one of them up walking often enough, I would knock on their door. "Roberto, get up. Get up! What are you doing?"

Roberto would moan and say, "I'm too tired. Keep inspiring us. You walk."

As a reporter, I am used to getting turned down. Instead, I'd argue with him from the doorway, "Man, you need to get up and move. Remember, fluid can build up in your lungs. Get up! You got this. You are in a cycle, and if you don't get up now it will be even tougher tomorrow. Get up!" Then I'd shuffle on to the next patient's room.

Sometimes, an administrator would come after me with a reminder that privacy laws meant I couldn't enter a patient's room. Next thing, there would be someone from the PR department asking what I was doing. Ha, ha—just being a reporter, always pushing my limits. Okay. I'm only *in* the doorway. It reminded me of the days of being told to leave an area because we couldn't cover a story and I would stand there and argue that we were on public property and it was my right. I believed that if I sat still in my room, I'd just wither away and die like so many others. I also believed that, as a well-educated reporter who researched the power of exercise and prehabilitation, I had an obligation to alert other patients. I couldn't look myself in the mirror if I didn't. Now, it brings me great joy to speak to patients and educate them about the power of prehabilitation.

CHAPTER 5

ArmorUp for LIFE® in Action/Discovery

> ArmorUp battle cry, becoming your own HERO, building your pit crew for success.

Fit to Fight

Dr. Levis's assurance echoed in my head: *"Your entire life, you prepared for this battle."* *"Your entire life, you prepared for this battle."* It became a mantra.

And indeed, I had. I'd kept fit and eaten clean, stayed engaged with my medical care once the cancer appeared, and knew how to fight like hell. I certainly put my Armor on. But I wasn't going to fight this battle by myself. It was time to turn my frustration into something positive—make an impact on how the healthcare system works and how patients are motivated, and save some lives along the way!

It was time for the ArmorUp for LIFE® battle cry, to put my armor on as my doctor said, and ArmorUp for LIFE®.

I rushed to flip open my laptop, with chemo still dripping through my IV. First, I typed out the hashtag #ArmorUp, and shared a post on social media creating fitness challenges: I would "ArmorUp" in the hospital and do all I could to be my fittest, if others would promise to do the same wherever they were. I wanted everyone to "Get fit to fight!"

I explained what I'd learned—that it's not a matter of *IF* but *WHEN* something will happen to us in our lifetime. It may not be COVID, it may not be cancer (chances are high—one in two men and one in three women will face some sort of cancer in his or her lifetime, according to the World Health Organization), but it will be something. And the better we prepare ourselves for those "someday" health crises, the greater the chance to survive.

And my own preparation—my years of running and working out—had empowered me to fight back against leukemia. I couldn't go train at the gym like I used to, but I could walk to prevent pneumonia, and to stay strong enough for treatment.

TAKEAWAY

"One day in bed will set you back four days in muscle strength, four days in bed will set you back an entire month," Dr. Levis had warned.

It worked!

Friends, fans, and warriors all over the country joined in and got moving to ArmorUp for whatever fight they'd face further down the road. And suddenly I had support. I didn't feel so alone and I felt like the journalist I had always been—the advocate to effect change on the world.

In the next days and weeks of treatment, with each hurdle I faced, I begged my friends on social media: "You ArmorUp for LIFE®, and I will do the same. *You* get out of bed to work out when the alarm goes off at 5:30 AM, even if you're tired and groggy, because you *can* and because you'll think of *my* fight. In exchange, I will walk the halls of the cancer unit, even when I feel I can't go any longer. We will hold each other accountable."

I urged my social media friends to start becoming their own heroes today. We posted our goals, and together made sure we followed through.

- You get up when the alarm goes off and work out, and I will ArmorUp for LIFE® and walk my laps.
- You take a dance class and ArmorUp for LIFE®, and I will get up and walk four times a day in the hospital.
- Make your green drink, and I'll make my smoothie.
- Get your rest, and I'll get mine.
- Start removing the stress out of your life, and I'll stay focused on fighting for mine.

In the world outside of a hospital, we think we have ideas about the qualities and markers that set us apart. The patients battling cancer on my floor were corporate executives, lawyers, engineers, pilots, accountants, radio DJs, housekeepers, teachers, construction workers, and waitresses. All from different walks of life.

As we have heard with COVID-19 time and time again, no matter who we were, how much money we made or didn't, we were in the same storm fighting an ugly disease with no official cure.

On the blood cancer unit, it didn't take long to realize the status quo no longer mattered.

Everybody had a cotton gown and a case number, a Hickman in their chest to feed chemo into the heart and precious little dignity. On the outside, shuffling through the halls, it appears not much sets you apart—not your car, your big house, your big contract. Not your grade point average or fancy degrees. Not your stock options, or prizes and awards. Status and who you are on the outside fade away. By the way, I wore bright workout clothes every single day. I wanted people to SEE me. . . to know I was alive. . . and I wanted to FEEL alive. I always said the minute you put those gowns on, you feel so defeated. That's why ArmorUp for LIFE® is working to help outfit cancer patients everywhere to ditch the gown and don fitness gear.

Our dreams were also the same. When our worlds collided with cancer and brought each of us to a dramatic pause, like COVID-19 did for so many, priorities shifted. We each wanted to go home to our kids and our families. We each wanted a second chance to live life again and do it differently. To spend more time with family, to be more aligned in our lives and careers and make more memories.

You know what went through my head? Regrets. Every single one of them.

I longed to have my freedom back—so I could do the things I didn't do when I was free to do them. I wanted to revisit each time my actions said *no* to things I wish I'd said *yes* to. I wanted to:

- Spend more time laughing and less time stressing out about things that, in the end, don't matter.
- Find balance in my career, to enjoy the now. Be fully present and not always have my head in social media.
- Focus more on *real* problems, not "first-world" problems.
- Be with friends and loved ones instead of working over-time, all the time.
- Go on vacation, instead of banking days of vacation.
- Make more memories with my husband and son.
- Visit family more often.

Tragically, not everybody got to do that. Dozens of friends I made at the hospital succumbed to this ugly disease. One by one I lost them. It was heartbreaking.

But while we were all in the same storm, I quickly learned we weren't all in the same boat. In the pandemic, the suffering for each family has differed. It's the same story for leukemia.

Beneath the gown and behind the masks, we each had a very different fight ahead. We didn't all start on the same playing field. We really weren't all in the same boat either.

Dr. Levis once pointed out, we all show up differently to the fight.

How well you've prepared for battle is what sets you apart. And because I showed up fit, I got a bigger bag of chemo, a stronger dose. They were able to push my limits. That's what gave me my second chance. It was no guarantee I would survive, but a guarantee that I would give myself the best chance possible.

> It is the same story that played out with how patients with COVID-19, just not with chemo.

If I had a 25 percent chance of survival, I wanted *ALL* 25, not a percentage less, and I vowed I was going to do all I could to make that happen. . . . Meet the medicine halfway, be an equal partner in my own success, and truly become my own HERO.

I sure didn't expect to go from medical reporter to patient and find myself on the other side of healthcare. But health crises can strike anyone, at any time. And let's get this clear, working out doesn't make you immune from illness; it prepares you. So please, fitness friends, you are not immune. You are not invincible. Now, my mission, and the mission of ArmorUp for LIFE®, is to inspire everyone to make the changes that will give him or her a second chance when it is needed.

Be well. Pre-habilitate. Prepare, Present, Prevail.

The Three ArmorUp for LIFE® Principles

During the COVID-19 pandemic, so many struggled to cope with the concept of staying at home. Fear, isolation, depression and loneliness spread as fast as the virus. I found myself sharing coping strategies during those troubling times.

To those who felt lost, I would remind them of my GPS strategies to get back on track and stay focused. Just like your phone's GPS can help you find your way, this GPS strategy can help you too!

TAKEAWAY

- Set a *Goal*
- Make a *Plan*
- Create a *Schedule*

Goals: I would set goals for each day. It started with a daily self-check in. Do I need help? Who can I ask to help me? How far can I walk today? When will I walk? How far to walk? Who to connect with? What projects can I work on that would bring me the most inner peace?

Plan: I decided to make a plan—always my strong suit. I would organize my cancer fight into a full-time job. SURVIVING WAS MY JOB. IT STILL IS. IT SHOULD BE YOURS. This would be no forty-hour-a-week job, though; I'd be on duty twenty-four hours a day, every single day. I scheduled down to the minute to keep me focused and busy: walking, eating, writing, virtual connections with Facetime and Zoom, doing research, making scrapbooks for Gabriel.

Schedule: Put it in writing, whether on the wall or on paper, and put down times and make yourself try to stick to it.

If I was going to live, a schedule was a must. I needed a routine. I put myself on a strict schedule, which I would adjust from day to day depending on my puking, diarrhea, nausea, MRSA staph infection, shingles, headaches and other side effects. Dr. Levis referred to these as petty torments, but even to this day they are anything but petty. But the schedule helped me push myself and say, "Oh wait. I'm late, it's time to walk." I do well with schedules, since newscasts are timed down to the minute. It's the only M.O. that I knew, so I thrived in it.

After my treatments were squared away each morning, this was my routine:

- 10:00 AM. Walk and talk to friends on my cell. I made lists of incoming phone calls I'd missed.
- 11:00 AM. Rest in my room.
- NOON. Lunch and write.
- 1:00 PM. Walk, outside if I could. I would take my IV stand—with a pouch of drugs hanging off the pole, connected to my Hickman valve—and roll it around the entire block, pushing it up the bumpy old cobblestone street. It must have looked pretty crazy, especially when I would time myself to see if I could beat my last lap—like when I was a runner. I was shuffling, not racing, but I would time my shuffles. I wanted to each time set a new PR (personal record), like most runners do. What was truly crazy-looking, though, were the smokers lining the sidewalks outside the hospital. Yes, smokers outside the cancer center. Including some hospital staff in uniform. More baffling: a bunch of the smokers were patients, hooked up to IVs for their cancer treatment at this

world-class institution. They were not meeting the medicine halfway. Even with my mask on, I'd have to hold my breath to pass by.

- 2:00 PM. Work on photo albums for Gabriel. In case I died, I wanted our son to remember how much I loved him. The psychologist on my pit crew had suggested it might be therapeutic, and it was.

- 3:00 PM. Do research for my Fox 7 story assignment, or continue work on the photo albums.

- 4:00 PM. This was my social hour. I'd walk through the hospital, eat at the cafe (I'd charge the expensive food they offered, but at least it was healthy), make friends, and informally interview patients to learn about how they ended up at Hopkins. It seems nearly everyone got there after being misdiagnosed somewhere else.

- 5:00 PM. Eat a snack and rest.

- 6:00 PM. Rest some more and do scrapbooking. It helped keep my mind occupied.

- 6:30 PM. FaceTime Gabriel! My little boy would be back at my mom's house after daycare and supper.

- 7:00 PM. Walk and cry. All day I worked hard to stay focused and positive, but by the end I could no longer hold back my emotion. Most of the other patients were sleeping; after their caregivers had headed home or were too busy with their own family members, I started to crumble. My loneliness became unbearable as I waited for Cesar to wrap up his long workday and drive from Bethesda. If I could, I'd walk a few laps around the floor. If I was really depressed, I would walk for hours, shedding the tears I'd saved up for my evening walk. I'd get my IV stand, attach a plastic bag with my wallet, puke tray, and phone, and roll out of my room wondering if anyone would notice if I never came back. I would cry and walk. Walk and puke. Cry for myself and my son. I covered every hallway in the entire Sydney Kimmel Cancer Center, and in the building connected to it.

- 9:00 PM. Finally, Cesar would arrive to stay the night on a makeshift bed in my room. My husband has always been amazingly stoic—I'll never understand how I managed to marry such a rock star. But his eyes looked hollow and glassy, and I could tell he was spent, numb. The very thing I craved most from him—his touch—we weren't to do. My body had no immune defenses, and any germs at all could kill me. *No one* could hug me or kiss me. And of course, the bustling newsroom where Cesar worked was chock full of microbes. Even holding my hand was a risk; because my blood system had very few platelets (which are responsible for clotting), any pressure could cause me to bruise or bleed. I was, for practical purposes, untouchable, living with cancer but dying of a broken heart at every turn. First thing, Cesar would wave to me, wash his hands, and put on a sterile yellow isolation gown. He would open up the reclining chair next to me, turn it into a bed, and kindly ask, "How was your day, Honey?" I would sob and stutter, wondering aloud if I'd be the next patient on the floor to die. All he could do was listen, tell me he loved me, and wait another hour or two for my routine.
- 10:00 PM blood draw, then go right to sleep.
- 11:00 PM. Sleep. Except it was never a full night's sleep— not even half. It was like a series of naps. There was the

Beep ... beep ... beep ... beep of the electronic chemo monitors as one bag of IV fluid finished and the next one started. Whenever I vomited, Cesar would sit up and help me. Take me into the shower to rinse off. By 2:00 AM. I'd be shivering and drenched in sweat from the medication. Nurses would come in to change the sheets on my bed. At 3:00 PM, I might wake up hallucinating, seeing cowboys in my room (yes, cowboys!), plus people coming to kill me. Around 4:00 AM, someone else would return to say my blood-draw results showed I was too low on red cells, then they would hook me up for a transfusion. Techs arrived about 4:30 AM to take my vitals: weight, temperature and blood pressure. And in between all the madness I would feel like I had a violent flu and puke. It never let up.

- 6:30 AM. Medical staff. A resident doctor would walk in and ask how the night went.
- 7:00 AM. Cesar would gently bathe me, then sneak in his own shower and dress for work. Technically, he wasn't allowed to use my bathroom because of infection risks, but the only other facility was a few buildings away, and he had neither time nor energy to get over there. He would trade his isolation gown for a fresh shirt, tie, dress pants, nice shiny shoes, and a smile, and then wait for rounds.
- 8:00 AM. Rounds. The daily assessment by the Hopkins team of doctors, residents, nurses, and researchers working on my case: They would literally form a circle outside my hospital room to confer. Together, these brilliant minds would consider the implications of the latest data

and adjust my treatment for the day. *Would I need another blood transfusion? More platelets? How best to treat my antibiotic-resistant staph infection? Should I be on isolation? If my breathing was slow, should they X-ray my lungs to check for fluids (possible pneumonia)? What's causing my persistent fever?*

Be Engaged—Have a Purpose

While doctors had their medical hats on, I had my reporter hat on . . . observing, researching, questioning every decision made. In my mind, I had a job to do, and not just for my own survival but to help those who may someday walk this path.

I treated those daily rounds like any news assignment I'd worked on as a TV journalist. What is my lead here? (The opening for viewers.) Are there other sides or perspectives to evaluate? Important context to add? What is the takeaway for viewers? How can this information in my update help them or someone they love?

Reporting my own case kept me busy. I asked questions, and I pushed doctors for answers. It's not enough to tell me what you are going to do—tell me why! What is your strategy? And what is it based on? How will this move affect me? Yep, I could hear my news director Pam thinking and asking these questions, back in Austin.

For my blog, I interviewed other patients on the hall to find out what drugs they were taking, what studies they were enrolled in (And why hadn't I been considered for that study?). As an anchor/reporter, if I wasn't picked for a choice assignment,

I would always ask why. I needed to understand the reasoning behind the decision, so I knew where I stood and what I might do better. In my new world, fighting cancer was no different.

Each day, I tried to find a takeaway for my audience, a key nugget of information that would have broad appeal to my followers on social media. A reason for them to care about my daily tribulations, and learn from them—perhaps even help spare a loved one from the same fate.

Once my weekly *story* was ready, I would upload it to Fox 7 in Austin to air on the morning show. That deadline Pam had given me kept me alive. It gave me a purpose and made me feel empowered. Isn't that what we all want? To know that what we are doing in our lives isn't in vain?

I remember the day she called to check on me and I was crying hysterically. I was losing my mind, staring at four walls in the hospital with no routine after the intense, round-the-clock structure of the news business. Journalists think about story angles every waking moment. And in broadcasting, on time means fifteen minutes early. Pam knew just what I needed. She offered, "if you want, let's run a story once a week. You make a schedule and I'll give you deadlines—but only if you are well enough, and only if you want to." It was the best distraction ever. This "assignment" on survival truly SAVED MY LIFE.

TAKEAWAY

If you know someone fighting for his or her life, give that person purpose, an assignment, a reason to keep living and it will change them.

Once the doctors had weighed in on my status and gave marching orders for the day, Cesar would blow me a kiss (over my mask) and head back to Bethesda, chin up and fears tucked away. He'd spend another long day **as** VP of NBC Sports Mid Atlantic, working to sustain his fragile family and our crucial health coverage. To this day, I don't know how my husband kept that brutal schedule and make it look seamless. He never took his eye off the ball at work. yet I knew he was there if I needed him.

I gave myself three main "assignments," which became the basis and core principles of ArmorUp for LIFE®:

- Meet the medicine halfway.
- Be an equal partner in your success.
- Become your own hero.

Let me explain.

Meet the Medicine Halfway

Doctors can't kill you trying to save you, so you have to do your part. Otherwise, they can't push the limits with aggressive treatment. Be strong enough for the strongest dose.

For me, that meant fully following through on my medical team's instructions—and then some. Those instructions included "don't get complacent," "don't give in," and "get up out of bed often to avoid fluid filling the lungs and leading to pneumonia." To make that happen, I knew that, for me, it included refusing *ALL* pain meds because I would rather be in pain than become a groggy version of myself and lose sight of my goals. My goal: Get out of bed to exercise as much as humanly possible, not just what was recommended.

It meant "presenting" my fittest self through careful attention to my diet (hint: hospital food isn't always as nutritious as you'd expect), trying to manage my stress, and minimizing pain medications—which blurred my mind and made it hard to focus.

By the way, I was so annoyed with the lack of options to eat clean and nutrient-dense food with minimal preservatives that one day I walked the halls looking for the office of the head of nutrition. I found him, and let him know my thoughts and concerns, like why is the protein shake loaded with sugar? Why do you offer artificial sweeteners here when there are studies linking them to cancer?

And it meant taking an active role in my treatment. Being sure I fully understood my disease and the options available to defeat it. And raising challenges when my intrepid research turned up questions. All this was second nature to a news reporter like me.

Be an Equal Partner in Your Success

Remove the noise around you and focus on the fight. Yes, your medical battle has to be your main focus. You can't be worrying about all the problems swirling around you that you're in no shape to take care of now. Wave the flag and get help.

This was an area of disappointment for me at the hospital. An area of "preparedness" a world-renowned institution lacked. It's called the whole patient approach. They needed to take into account the psycho-oncology of treatment. I'm not talking about just acknowledging that patient outcomes and success also rely on emotional well-being and ability to be fully in the game, but provide a support system for that well-being. They didn't. It was a HUGE void. So, I had to figure out a strategy on my own.

For me, that meant identifying anything and everything standing in the way of what I—and my family—needed to survive this ordeal. And there was a loooong list, things you could never imagine. The hospital just wasn't set up to handle so many parts of my struggle.

Then it meant asking for help and accepting it. I had to rely on friends, family, associates, and perfect strangers to pull resources together. That was hard, since I was proud of being pretty self-sufficient. But I had to admit I couldn't do it all myself.

Become Your Own Hero

Don't count on everyone to save you. Put the work in to save yourself. Don't lie down and surrender. Get up and fight. Somehow, gather up the inner resources to push through this hellish new reality and *prevail*.

For me, that meant staying strong and positive. Which is how I'd always lived my life. But I'd never faced anything like this.

It meant having a mission and a purpose—long known to be so crucial to healing and resilience. My new mission was spreading the message of ArmorUp for LIFE®. My purpose, above all, was surviving to see my son grow up.

And it meant, in the worst times, putting faith over fear.

Meet the medicine halfway. Be an equal partner in my success. Become my own hero. That was my job now, and I dove into it with hope and all the energy I could muster.

> This is the same strategy you must apply if and when you are diagnosed with an illness, whether it's COVID-19, cancer, heart disease, Lyme, or anything else.

Building Your Pit Crew

I set about giving doctors their fittest possible patient. I had the *walking* part down cold, of course. I shuffled through the halls, rolling my IV stand alongside, for countless miles. I walked when I had fevers. I walked and puked as I struggled from the chemo side effects of nausea. I always got back up and kept going. I took the dozens of medications they prescribed; this is just a sampling of the forty plus medications I took during my treatment.

- Cytarabine 2000 mg/m2 continuous infusion over three days
- Etoposide 400 mg/m2/day x three days
- Daunorubicin 45 mg/m2/day x three days

- Cytarabine 3000 mg/m2/day for six doses over five days
- Bone marrow transplant: Fludarabine 30 mg/m2/day x five days, cyclophosphamide 14.5 mg/kg/day x 2 days, TBI 200 CGy, cyclophosphamide 60 mg/kg/day x two days
- Pomalidomide for several weeks
- Voriconazole for several months
- Moxifloxacin for several months
- Tacrolimus

Most of them came through the Hickman from a drip (the chemo toxins stung my veins). Others I had to swallow in pill or liquid form depending on if I was suffering from a very painful condition called mucositis. That's when I couldn't swallow or even sip a straw so it was given through IV.

I took pain meds, briefly—at first. But I quickly realized I couldn't co-exist with pain meds and achieve my goals. They knocked me out. I could have a pill whenever I needed, unless it was too soon for the next dose. But the few times I took one, I'd wake up exhausted, not wanting to move or even sit up. I was too groggy to function, let alone go walking. I grew more depressed and fearful. It fed a vicious cycle that I knew would lead to my death, like others I had lost. I couldn't afford that, even if it meant tremendous suffering.

I made the decision to refuse pain pills unless I was in dire agony. Staying fit, engaged, and not groggy was more important to my survival than not hurting (as much), I figured.

Instead, I signed up to participate in a study on medical massage and *Reiki*. It was only fifteen minutes a week. It helped me, though the sessions were never long enough. But I knew the trade-off and pay-off long-term from massage. I witnessed it. Eventually, with donated gifts, I was able to hire massage therapists to come to the hospital to treat my pain and anxiety — and it worked!

I was getting awe-inspiring, world-class treatment from my medical team, so I was surprised to find that the food available to us wasn't up to that standard. When I couldn't handle solids, they'd offer Popsicles loaded with sugar — a real no-no, in my eyes, for cancer patients. There are many studies that show that sugar actually feeds cancer. The meal-replacement drinks contained a long list of ingredients deemed unhealthy by many studies. Even the regular saltine crackers that might offset nausea and vomiting were off-limits to me, because I'm gluten-intolerant.

I rarely ordered hospital food. I gave money to friends, other caregivers on the hall, and even nurses who kindly (and secretly) added items to their shopping list to get foods I knew would help fuel me and my body for success: avocados, nuts and whole-fruit organic icepops (the snack shop down in the lobby sold these). Nothing processed. Nothing with sugar. Later, I brought my Vitamix blender from home to make nutrient-dense shakes for myself and other patients — exactly what our bodies needed!

I researched my disease online, and learned everything I could about treating it. This is where being a healthcare reporter worked in my favor. Not because I had the answers — I just knew how to ask the questions. I approached every single day in treatment like a news story and an investigation.

Observing, researching, questioning and pushing for answers, I found startling statistics from the World Health Organization and other researchers.

- One of every three women, and one of every two men, will face cancer in his or her lifetime.
- During chemotherapy treatment, the more you walk, the better your chance of survival.
- Patients who don't get out of bed risk dying of pneumonia even before cancer kills them.
- Stress can cause inflammation; inflammation is a fertilizer for cancer.

I asked tough questions of my doctors. Why does exercise matter? Why are so many people dying around me? Was I going to die? (I asked this one every single day.) Why did I need a certain treatment? Why was a certain drug not being offered? Why wasn't a particular research/trial drug offered to me? Why are my eyes on fire?

The more I learned, the more I shared in the weekly news reports I filed from my bedside. I wanted every patient to have the tools for success. Spreading the word—both on social media and in weekly segments I filed for my Fox station in Austin— kept me motivated.

Trust me, I was meeting the medicine halfway, and then some. This is something you need to ask yourself today, long before you fall ill.

Long before you fall ill, know who is in your pit crew and what role each person will play to successfully lead you to the finish line.

This was a lesson I learned after I witnessed my first NASCAR race in Dallas, on one of my very first assignments in the Lone Star State. I was in awe of how this team worked together to successfully help the driver get to the finish line and win.

From the minute I covered the story. . . that image was forever etched in my memory. I would go on to cover NASCAR extensively, along with football and other Texas staples throughout my next ten years in the Lone Star State.

- What can you do today to meet the medicine halfway?
- Are you truly doing your part? If you get cancer or something else today, would you get the small bag of chemo or the large?
- If you get COVID, how prepared are your lungs?

There is no one-size-fits-all treatment for illness. You present well, you get a stronger dose. End of story.

My first time at the speedway I remember the pitched and curvy track, the crowd full of proud Texas accounts, the whine of the high-tech engines blurring by, the smell of fuel and rubber. I loved it, but I was awestruck when I saw a pit crew work its magic.

In that low, low moment, a memory came to me and I decided *everyone* needed a "pit crew" to fight cancer. This really goes for any illness or crisis.

Before you suit up for your next drive, let me explain.

Of course, each car had a driver behind the wheel, risking life and limb for victory. But that wasn't the half of it. Whenever someone pulled into the "pit" beside the track to refuel, a human machine of specialists would swarm over every inch of the vehicle. In seconds—*seconds*—they'd flip that road-hard race car back into a roaring piece of competition.

Everyone on the crew had a role: Two or three or four swapped the tires, others gushed fuel into the tank, mechanics made safety checks, and somebody cleaned the windshield while the driver soaked up a sports drink and strategy tips. Every movement was choreographed like a dance, no movement wasted. It was a miracle of teamwork, and I never tired of watching. It wasn't a tribe. . . just surrounding you with comfort. It was a pit crew. A team invested in your success.

I had to put that concept into motion each day at the hospital as I was also overcome with worry. Sometimes, it crowded out everything else. Would I live? How could we ever pay for this, even with insurance coverage? Would Gabriel be traumatized? My mother was having a nervous breakdown. Who could help my seventy-year mother care for my son? Was Cesar's job safe? Would I ever work again? Why was I so depressed?

I was used to managing everything solo, more or less: career, baby son, long-distance marriage, a household, an active life. And I'd been juggling all those arrangements, keeping all the balls in the air. Now everything was crashing down, and it was all I could do to fight for my life. I felt helpless.

In fact, I came to realize, it was a lot like the newsrooms I'd worked in. Sure, when I finally became an anchor, I got to be the face of the station—and the network—but I *never* could have done it all by myself. My ability to deliver the news depended on the support of dozens of others. There were brilliant and talented producers, news directors, cameramen, sound engineers, programmers, prompters, designers, lighting and makeup artists, film editors, network coordinators—and all those "business-side" people who kept the lights on and the broadcast license current.

They only made it look effortless for me to do my job well. Like a pit crew.

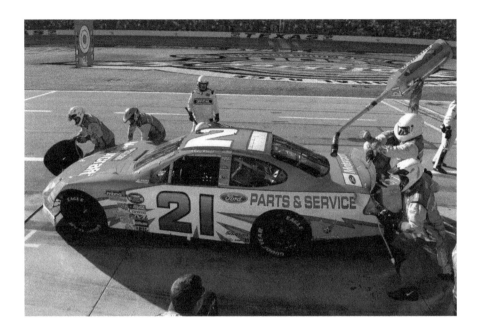

Image by Skeeze from Pixabay

Well, now I desperately needed my own pit crew. I was trying to race to a victory over cancer, but all the wheels had come off and I was running on empty.

On my computer, I created a spreadsheet. In the rows and columns, I listed:

- Each and every problem that was getting in the way of my success—urgent needs, including childcare, mental health help, legal problems like a will and guardianship paperwork and financial issues, and diet challenges.

- The name of every single person who had reached out to offer help since my diagnosis—friends, family, viewers, social media connections.
- Skills and resources that each of those people might be able to provide, trying to imagine the most effective way they could support me.

It was quite a revelation! I had an incredible community on my side, even if many of those in my pit crew-to-be had never met each other.

Now came the hard part; asking them for help. My pride sure didn't like the idea. It wasn't like me to expect to be rescued. But then I thought, *if a winning NASCAR driver depends on a pit crew to succeed, then why can't I?*

What is wrong with getting help? What is wrong with being led to the finish line by a team that's invested in my success?

"Nothing."

Plus, I would do anything to live and watch my son grow up! At that point, I knew I would have to surrender to reach my goal.

I was also never so thankful that, throughout my entire career, I had put so much good out into the world by way of volunteering for so many great organizations and people. The good was about to come back to me ten-fold.

TAKEAWAY

GIVE and you will get back. Your good will multiply when you least expect it.

So, using my spreadsheet, I contacted these generous friends to enlist them onto my pit crew, and called each of them back with a specific plan for his or her role in my success. Most well-intentioned people are baffled about what to give cancer patients, so they just send random gifts. My pit crew approach took care of that dilemma!

Some donated money. Some donated time. Some donated professional expertise or special skills. The help I needed came pouring in.

"I can't visit, but I can lead an online fundraiser to help you pay your bills," said Alice Alston from Austin.

Janice Caprelian, my long-time friend and my son's god-mother, volunteered, "I have airline points to use, so I will fly in to help unpack your house in Virginia."

Natali Ceniza, a long-time friend in Atlanta who actually hired me at CNN lived near my mom, and offered to help with Gabriel's childcare. "I can pay for it, or drive over to check on what your mom needs."

Amy Katzenberg is a digital strategist I'd met in Austin, skilled in web development and branding and being an amazing listener and friend. "Let me build you a website, develop your ArmorUp for LIFE® logo, and give you a platform for your voice to be heard. Then you will have something to focus on and a way to help others through your story," she offered. That was huge. And looking forward to my brief visits home between rounds of chemo, she also picked up the tab for a monthly house-cleaning service, so I could just focus on being reunited with my family.

Incredible Austin colleagues Drex and Michele Graham, who own Bounce Marketing, said they'd help design ArmorUp for LIFE® banners and do other promotions for the project.

I knew Todd Wallace from NBC in Dallas. He was my co-anchor and a very spiritual friend. He and his wife would link up over FaceTime to pray with me.

Dr. Allison Chase is a child psychologist and Fox news contributor I'd worked with in Austin. She offered her time on the phone with me—what a blessing! She gave me the mental health help and guidance I wasn't getting in the hospital. She listened, answered my questions, and taught me coping tools.

Tracey Garcia, the friend who held my hand on that first, scary day I arrived at Johns Hopkins, visited every two weeks. She did my makeup to make me feel beautiful, brought me home-cooked meals, and took my laundry back with her.

When I told my new Virginia friend Tracy Parent about how rigid and uncomfortable my hospital bed was, she ordered up a much-needed memory-foam pillow.

Two nursing students at Johns Hopkins, Susannah and Geny, both from Austin, heard about my plight and began stopping by my room each day on the way to class. They'd give me foot massages, and they even bought a twin comforter to replace the cold, thin blankets on my bed. More angels!

I knew Kristi and Eddie Rodriquez from our new neighborhood in VA. Not only did they donate money to my fundraiser, they went shopping for walking sneakers that would help me keep moving safely. Kristi and Eddie showed up at the hospital with *nine*, yes NINE, pairs of shoes for me to try on!

And my Fox 7 community in Austin came through big-time. Colleagues sent me fitness workout gear.

But news director Pam Vaught, who is also my friend, will never know how important a role she played in my survival. I called her one night in a complete meltdown, screaming, crying and losing it. I was worried I was going to die. I was worried I was going to stare at those four walls and die of a broken heart. How she responded *saved my life*. I want to repeat that—how she responded saved my life. She gave me work. She gave me purpose.

TAKEAWAY

If you know someone who is struggling to fight and is losing hope, give them an assignment, give them purpose, make them feel obligated to you so they have an obligation to commit to living and not surrendering to dying.

It was Pam who got to know me during the ten years I worked for her. She knew my work ethic. She knew what made me tick and what gave me drive. She understood that I needed a voice and a purpose, so she assigned me stories to do from the hospital. She took my struggle and made me see how it's *everyone's* struggle, giving me more determination to fight and live so I could help others.

The list of members in the bad-ass pit crew I built goes on and on. But each one played a pivotal role in my survival, working to remove the noise and worry so I could focus on my fight. Although I rarely had visitors and was far away from my most familiar support system, my pit crew made me feel part of a team, and never alone. It made getting through a hellish ordeal manageable.

I was an equal partner in my success.

I share this detailed list with you so you can use it to generate ideas of WHO would be in your pit crew. Who could help you in times of need? As you witnessed with COVID, patients need a lot of help and support and, much like me, it was from afar and all last-minute. Thinking of your pit crew? Build it now to utilize later.

TAKEAWAY

Who is in YOUR pit crew? Who can you assign jobs to? Can you make a list and reach out to people who can help?

Be Your Own Hero and Push Through

Somehow, we each have to gather up the inner resources to push through this hellish new reality and *prevail*. For me, that meant staying strong and positive. Which is how I'd always lived my life. But I'd never faced anything like this. It meant having a mission and a purpose—long known to be so crucial to healing and resilience. My new mission was spreading the message of ArmorUp for LIFE®. My pivot became my purpose, above all—surviving to see my son grow up.

And it meant, in the worst times, putting faith over fear.

I was becoming my own hero.

I was Armoring Up for LIFE.

CHAPTER 6

Getting Prepared

Your body is preparing every single day for illness, whether you like it or not. Your actions each and every day play a crucial role in how you actually show up for illness. You can take an active role and sit in the driver seat or sit back and do nothing. The choice is yours.

Each and every day you are laying the groundwork and foundation for *how* you show up to your illness, whatever it may be and whenever it will happen. You are preparing *your* body for how you present to your medical team. You have to go beyond the mask and think about how you are going to prepare your body for illness. I don't have a choice about wearing a mask, given my immune system, but regardless where you stand on the mask issue, my question to you is . . . what are you doing to do beyond the mask to get your body prepared for illness? The mask won't prepare you for COVID or cancer, heart disease or any other illness. You have to take those steps.

What steps are you taking on your own to reduce the inflammation that leads to illness so you can present as a stronger patient?

What steps are you taking to boost your immune system so you can fight better?

Remember, it is not about the skinny jeans. That won't make you stronger.

And later on in this chapter, I will address why I'm a firm believer in mixing Eastern and Western medicine.

First, let's think about how often we throw around the term Rehab. You have knee or back surgery and you, of course, go to REhab. It's a priority. Shoulder surgery? REhab. Breast cancer surgery? REhab to move your arms over your head again. Surgery. REhab. In each case, it's a no-brainer to go. It's actually part of the program that is offered. Surgery + Rehab. It is how you recover properly. You have a drug problem? You go to REhab. Eating Disorder? REhab. Depression and mental and emotional issues that get escalated? REhab.

Where the hell is PREhab? Why isn't this part of the program and pushed as hard as we push REhab?

When was the last time your doctor, physician's assistant, or nurse said: "Okay, so we have your surgery scheduled—let's get you prepared. Let's PREhab!"

Or

"You have cancer. Here's how you can PREhab for your upcoming surgery, chemo, and radiation."

OR

"Does your insurance company offer a program to PREhab?"

Not often enough and not in this way.

It *SHOULD* be part of the program. A wheel of success.

PREhab + treatment + REhab = better outcomes.

Again, you are preparing each and every day, surgery or not, for an illness that will come your way. It will happen, like it or not. Sometime in your lifetime you will face *some* sort of illness, and *how* you prepare today will play a role in how you *present*. How strong a dose of treatment can you physically handle? How will you get through it and come through the other side of it? Think about most of the patients affected by the coronavirus. The more fit they went into it, the better they came out. Why? As my world-renowned leukemia doctor once said, "We can't kill you trying to save you."

He later explained, "If your heart isn't strong enough, blood pressure isn't good enough, weight isn't good enough, lungs aren't fit enough, we have to drop your dose. We can only give you what you can physically handle." But I want to break this down even more.

The Five Pillars to PREhabilitation to ArmorUp for LIFE®

What I learned in my year of hospitalization and hell was that there are five ways to PREPARE or PREhab for illness long before you ever fall ill. The obvious is getting physically prepared, but there are actually five pillars to PREhabilitation to ArmorUp for LIFE®. It is a pillar of success. You need all five of them:

1. Diet
2. Exercise
3. Lifestyle
4. Spirituality
5. Financial

I will break these out in a moment.

First, let's talk about why lack of preparedness is an issue and why so many of us put "PREhabbing" off.

In my search for answers, I would press Dr. Levis to tell me more. He is not only brilliant but fascinating.

How patients present is our biggest issue.

For example, perhaps you notice chest tightness or tingling in your arms over recent weeks. Maybe it's headaches. You are stressed. You're more tired than usual or maybe you are just short on patience and biting everyone's heads off at home or the office. For me, I started noticing my stomach was swollen. I was exhausted, had swollen lymph nodes, some bruises. I found ways to justify each and every issue. You do too. You write it off, you discount it, you deny it because that light was flickering and then it went away.

The issue is, we don't collectively look at our problems from a whole-patient approach.

Second, we discount the symptoms and convince ourselves they are nothing so we can go about our busy day. Instead, we let them fester. The mentality is we will "fix" X, Y, and Z when the problem comes up another time. We don't have time to prepare. We are too busy. It's not a priority. It's not scary enough. "People need me." "My schedule is too tight." Other things on our schedule are WAYYYYYYY too important. I have to go here; I have to go there, and it can wait. So, we wait until it gets bad enough that it's urgent and then we try to fix it. We wait for the problem to be so bad that we simply have no choice but to say fix me now!

It's like pulling up to an auto repair shop after driving your car into the ground, blowing past every maintenance light, ignoring those flickering check engine lights and any odd noises until it is "convenient" and fits into your schedule. Then when the car stops, the brakes go, you rush to the auto shop and want what you did over a year's time to get fixed *now* . . . like right now . . . and fast. Yes! It's the mechanic's job to fix the car! But *you* drove it into the ground! Did you do *any* maintenance? Did you change the oil on time?

Most of us have done this at some point in our lives. *This* is how we treat our bodies.

For leaders this happens all the time; work piles up, and "self-care" often takes a back seat (like that warning light) to other "pressing" priorities. It did for me.

But here's a newsflash for you. The hospital or doctor's office isn't an overnight repair shop. You *must* meet the medicine halfway.

Sadly now, in the midst of the COVID-19 crisis, the world has stopped turning on its axis. Now you actually have the time to listen to your body. Listen to any warning lights that were or are going off. But you can't do anything about it because the resources are being over-allocated to COVID-19 treatments and you can't go to the doctor. You may have even self-reflected and kicked yourself thinking, why did I not go when I had the chance? That was me, staring at four walls battling leukemia for a year. I had so much time to self-reflect. I played over and over in my head every single missed opportunity to seek medical attention for issues I simply wrote off.

Your job is to learn how you can meet the medicine halfway. Your job is to step back and look at the big picture. Do a total body assessment, list what ailments you have, get a physical with blood work, and then make a game plan. A basic CBC (complete blood count) detected my leukemia. Now, even more sophisticated tests are available to look at genetic markers and raise other red flags. Seek them out. Get them done.

I get it. You think you are taking the right steps. I did too. But I also easily wrote off various warning signs and looked at them as independent from the other issues. You have to look at yourself as a whole patient. So does your medical team. Problems don't always fester in silos.

Pre-cancer, I thought I was meeting the medicine halfway. I drank the green drinks. Checked off the fitness box with tough workouts and hot yoga. Juiced. Cut the gluten, dairy, sugar, and caffeine from my diet. I thought I had all my bases covered. EXCEPT SLEEP. Deep, restorative sleep. Eventually, the wheel fell off the bus, as I like to say. Sleep is part of the wheel of success for total well-being. Not just any sleep. Deep sleep. I was also chronically stressed.

The genius of ArmorUp for LIFE® is, you have the chance today to become your own HERO.

So, let's break down those five pillars.

Diet (Elevate your plate during times of stress)

This is a big one. I saw it in TV newsrooms daily. I would hear "I don't have time to eat." I even hear this from my husband and oftentimes when I would coach people on their diets. It was the justification to just grab anything and go. You're busy. I get it.

"I don't have time! I have too much on my plate." Yes, except food! So, you either eat junk or skip meals, when actually, these times of stress are when you need to eat clean (fewer preservatives, sugars, unhealthy fats, etc.) to fuel your body for success. Research shows the rise and fall of blood sugars, like from junk food, can set the stage for diabetes.

I had the honor of having dinner one evening with cancer researchers. I looked around the table and noticed every single person was eating a plant-based meal. My eyes opened up. What are the odds? All of them? The curious reporter in me asked, "Are all of you plant-based?"

The gentleman next to me said, "Yes and no. During times of high level of stress and demanding hours for a project." He added, "We know our lifestyle is going to add to the stress in our bodies and the inflammation that is detrimental, so we control what we can and switch to a plant-based diet during exhausting projects. When the projects are over, we move to a more modified healthy diet but we treat ourselves to other foods we love."

I thought, *Wow! How great, and what a great approach we can all learn from.* It makes perfect sense—switch to plant-based and up your clean eating strategy during times of stress to give your body what it needs to succeed.

You can't put Kool-Aid in your car because you are in a hurry and think it will run, right? It needs the *right* fuel. You can't put junk in your body and think it will perform at its highest level.

Let Food Be Thy Medicine

Since ancient times, many cultures have used food for medicine. It is and can be your medicine. I'm always baffled that we all don't heed this advice more often. Ancient Chinese medicine uses food for medicine. It has worked for thousands of years. Yes, we need Western medicine, but what is wrong with having Eastern medicine complement it with good food choices that have anti-inflammatory, anti-viral, anti-fungal properties and more?

Consider going plant-based on certain days to help decrease the inflammation you might be adding to your body with your lifestyle. Fruits and vegetables are anti-inflammatory. There are amazing meals you can create that are full of flavor and packed with nutrients (I'll share a few recipes in the back of the book). Remove the processed, fatty, and fried foods, and make healthier swaps. Add spices and flavors that are beneficial to your body and its healing.

In Ayurvedic medicine there are many spices used in the effort to promote healing. You can make your own mix of those spices, which include ginger, cumin, coriander, fennel, cardamom, and (the big one) turmeric. Ayurvedic medicine suggests you take 1/2 teaspoon with every meal. You can find countless Indian recipes that include these spices.

There have been countless studies showing the benefits of turmeric and its cancer-fighting properties. In fact, the National Institutes of Health (NIH) even has an entire page on its website detailing the many studies that are looking at how curcumin (the active ingredient in turmeric) is found to potentially stop the growth of tumor cells by blocking some of the enzymes needed for cell growth. It may help to decrease or prevent certain cancers.

Why not find ways to incorporate curcumin into your diet? But instead of just popping a turmeric pill, try picking some up at the store and add it to your meals (https://www.cancer.gov/about-cancer/treatment/clinical-trials/intervention/curcumin).

Again, let your food choices work with you and not against you. Let food be thy medicine.

Think this is crazy? You don't have time to meal prep and make meals or snacks like this? I share this with leaders all the time. If you can't take care of you, how can you take care of your team or anyone else? You do strategic planning at work, right? You do this in so many aspects of your life—car insurance, life insurance, even retirement. So why is your company's bottom line often more important than your own?

Most of the time during treatment we aren't up for big meals. Our taste buds change; they become very metallic, and what we once loved no longer tastes good and can even gross us out. One day you love it and the next day it will make you gag. I discovered that the food offered in the "pantry" was loaded with sugar, preservatives, and ingredients I couldn't pronounce and my body couldn't break down on a good day, let alone while I was at my lowest and fighting for my life. I needed food to help me ArmorUp for LIFE® and meet the medicine halfway. I needed food to help me put my best foot forward. Foods like these:

- **Organic WHOLE FRUIT Popsicles**
  Sadly, the only Popsicles offered on the hall are all sugar. The cheapest Popsicles around. As you know, there are many studies that sugar feeds cancer.

- **Homemade Granola**
  A great nutrient-dense and clean-eating snack, high in protein and good carbs!

- **Organic Fruit**

  Note: Some oncology units allow fresh fruit during treatment, others do not. The concern is the risk of bacteria for a patient when he/she has no immune system. When you have no immune system, it could just take one infection to spike a fever and lead to tragic consequences.

- **Organic plant-based meal replacement drinks**

- **Gluten-Free crackers and snacks**

  I am gluten-free, but I believe it's a good option for anyone undergoing chemo. Chemo affects the gut, and gluten is believed to be hard on the gut. I loved my GF crackers.

- **Vitamix drinks**

  I brought my Vitamix to my hospital room. I made my own meal replacement drinks. I was able to clean out the machine in the pantry. There was no way I was drinking that Ensure drink.

Exercise

Fitness matters. Get MOVING! Stay MOVING!

Every day when you wake up, think to yourself, *How fit am I to fight an illness?* Could you suit up for battle and face COVID or cancer? Find something you can do each day to improve your health. Go on a walk, take a run, or do some yoga; take up dancing, golf, swimming or some sort of movement. Post COVID-19, you can find nearly any workout online. You don't need money; you need discipline to get fit. Trust me, you will need discipline to survive. Start working on it. Movement matters. It will improve your cardiovascular health. It will help your heart. Strengthen your lungs. Build your muscle strength and prepare your body for illness both mentally and physically.

There are countless studies on the impact of exercise and preparing for illness. For example, we do know that exercise slows down the release of stress hormones in our bodies and we know that stress (chronic stress) is what has been known to cause inflammation in the body. If that is not enough to convince you to get up and start moving, perhaps this statement from the chair of the Clinical Oncology Society of Australia Exercise and Care Group will.

"If we could turn the benefits of exercise into a pill it would be demanded by patients, prescribed by every cancer specialist and subsidized by government—it would be seen as a major breakthrough in cancer treatment."

The Clinical Oncology Society of Australia brought together twenty health organizations to create a position statement saying: "Exercise is to be embedded as part of standard practice in cancer care and to be viewed as an adjunct therapy that helps counteract the adverse effects of cancer and its treatment." COSA adds now in its guidelines that withdrawing from exercise after diagnosis or while undergoing treatment actively harms cancer patients' chances of survival. Studies show chemo works better if you exercise. I walked and puked with fevers, and I cried, but I never gave up. Plus, once the doctors told me that pneumonia can take you before cancer does, it was on. I never sat still. When you lie down you risk allowing fluid to collect in your lungs which can lead to pneumonia . . . another reason to get up and ArmorUp for LIFE®.

So many people from around the globe reached out to me and asked how they can help cancer patients. Here is a list of gifts I suggested. It is also the list of items ArmorUp for LIFE® has handed out to cancer patients.

- Fitness tracker
- Sneakers/tennis shoes to walk
- Socks
- Athletic wear (easy to access with a catheter or to take on/off, like a sweatshirt with a zipper)Women's jogging bras or children's tanks (easy for unexpected MRI's)
- Women's and men's underwear (hospital disposable ones are horrible!)
- Robes
- Workout tops (sleeveless)
- Pants (yoga types)
- Hand weights or exercise bands. I used hand weights at times but it all depends on where the catheter (Hickman or PICC line to run the chemo) is placed. You can't put pressure by lifting weights. This is a decision the doctors need to agree on.
- Flip flops—for using in the room to protect you from germs on the floor

Lifestyle

Think about your life and the toxicity surrounding it. Covid-19 and the pandemic gave you plenty of time to self-reflect. Odds are you realized how much stress was in your life. Now the work is figuring out where and how to cut it down or cut it out. Not just the stress in your job, but the toxicity you allow into your life and in your relationships. Stress levels matter.

For most of us the diet and exercise might be easy to check off, but it's the lifestyle that gets us. It's what got me. I was waking up at 1:45 AM to go into work. Working until one, two, or three in the afternoon depending on breaking news. Then I'd care for a newborn until 9:00 or 10:00 PM and then repeating that cycle. No break. No recharge. No sleep.

Stress and sleep deprivation greatly impact your total body health.

It should scare you as much as eating bad food and missing a workout—but we don't seem to take it as seriously.

One doctor told me:

"You can have the best diet in the world, drink all the green drinks you want, and exercise, but if you aren't sleeping . . . you aren't regenerating new cells . . . you are inviting problems."

Sleep restores the building blocks of the body. Not just *ANY* sleep. Deep sleep.

You might think that prioritizing your well-being is too hard. It's not convenient . . . it doesn't pay the bills . . . right? It keeps getting pushed down the priority list when "WORK" gets in the way . . .

Well, I'm here to tell you the GENIUS of ArmorUp is that you have the chance to "BECOME YOUR OWN HERO" —TODAY.

ArmorUp IS ABOUT ANYONE.

Because life always punches us from our blindside. And my fight and recovery have some important lessons:

- No matter how much you prevent, you MUST still PRE-PARE because something will happen.
- Maybe it's not cancer—but it will be something . . .

Why?

- Stress is an American killer
- *Everyone, please own this*
- Success should not kill us

BUT. . .

- When we don't prioritize our own well-being
- When we don't put the oxygen mask on ourselves so we can be better to those dependent on us
- When we don't check out the warning light
- We are playing with FIRE

Why?

- Stress sabotages the immune system
- Chronic stress causes inflammation in the body
- Inflammation, as we learn from countless studies, is a fertilizer for cancer

One of my favorite studies is from Carnegie Mellon:

- https://www.pnas.org/content/early/2012/03/26/1118355109.abstract
- http://www.psy.cmu.edu/people/cohen.html

- https://www.cmu.edu/homepage/health/2012/spring/
  stress-on-disease.shtml

I found that when our systems are constantly bathed in cortisol (the stress hormone released when we are scared or pushing ourselves through a big project) and we don't recharge and restore cells, our body loses the ability to regulate inflammation and *BOOM*.

The flood gates open for illness . . .

Another study talks about the impact of stress:

- https://www.ncbi.nlm.nih.gov/pmc/articles/
  PMC3037818/?utm_source=yahoo-food&utm_medium
  =referral&utm_campaign=content-partnerships

Stress might promote cancer indirectly by weakening the immune system's anti-tumor defense or by encouraging new tumor-feeding blood vessels to form.

This study shows that stress hormones, such as adrenaline, can directly support tumor growth and spread. Cancer cells have come up with a way to bypass cell death and to break off from tumors, spread throughout the body (in blood or other fluid) and form new tumors at distant sites—the study found that stress influences so many normal physiological processes. Why wouldn't it be involved in tumor progression?

Yes, stress can kill you. Stress can land you on the other side of healthcare.

It did for me.

When you go days and days without sleep because of a work project, staffing issue, a budget deadline, a problem at home with the kids and family… I get it. Life happens. But you must pull over, regroup and refuel. You must maintain the car. No, you don't have to refuel for the exact amount of time you were missing sleep, but you have to fill up the tank. You MUST hit that reset button.

You can start with a few simple steps:

- Take out your phone. Put in your calendar "ArmorUp for LIFE®" (or "Workout," "Me time," or whatever word you choose) and put it on repeat. Let this serve as a visual reminder each day to refuel and restore. Trust me, when you actually have to move it and you notice you are deleting it daily, you will have a reality check that you are not ArmoringUp for LIFE®.
- Schedule your own doctor appointments for your own tests. Physicals, blood work etc.
- Set goals, drink plenty of water. Ditch the soda, cut the sugar, cut the artificial sweeteners.
- Take the steps, walk the extra lap—are you sitting when you could be standing?
- Take time to meditate. Find a meditation app or find a yoga studio.

An Everest College Survey found some startling statistics:

- 83% of US workers are stressed
- Stress results in as much as $300 billion in lost productivity
- 60% to 80% of workplace accidents result from *stress*
- 1,000,000 employees miss work each day because of stress

Source: Everest College Survey, Health Advocate, ComPsych

Everest College study link for sourcing

https://everestcollege.wordpress.com/2013/06/10/83-of-americans-are-stressed-out-at-work/

Stress and its Impact on the Body

The stress and toxicity of your lifestyle will impact how well you present. Let's face it. Stress is going to happen. It's inevitable. But what kind of stress and how long you allow it to dominate your life is what matters. Whether it is our high-pressured jobs, the stress of a pandemic, depression and loneliness, or busy traffic that keeps your body in that perceived threat mode and chronic stress, staying in that state of intense stress for too long is a problem.

As I shared earlier, when you get stressed over and over again and it becomes chronic, that will take a toll on your immune system and as a result make you more susceptible to illness. And as they say in sports, the best defense is a good offense. That includes ArmoringUp for LIFE® with relaxation response strategies such as breathing techniques and yoga.

During the relaxation response, the body moves toward a state of physiological relaxation, where blood pressure, heart rate, digestive functioning, and hormonal levels return to normal levels. When you start to breathe faster that should be your cue that you're unconsciously holding onto it. That's the very stress that will start to take a toll on your health and your nervous system. It sure took a toll on my health.

My life before cancer was a constant state of stress and breaking news. As I shared with you before, I NEVER came down to refuel. Even as a dedicated yogi, I would sneak my phone into the class and I'm embarrassed to share I would wait for the right posture to come up for me to tap my phone, check a message and sneak out so I didn't miss the big story.

Now, the phone is off. I am fully present. My body can fully relax. I know the difference. I *feel* the difference.

The steps you take to effectively manage it and essentially work to counteract it or (at least limit the damage) will matter, according to this Harvard study: https://www.health.harvard.edu/mind-and-mood/relaxation-techniques-breath-control-helps-quell-errant-stress-response

Your exhale is directly tied to relaxation response in the brain. When you don't have that relaxation response because you are breathing too hard, you're in that state of stress. Managing stress through breathing is an excellent way to meet the medicine halfway. This is how you take steps to be part of the solution and become your own HERO.

Yoga is Medicine

Yoga is certainly medicine for the soul and for the immune system. It is a mind-body practice that is considered one of many types of complementary and integrative health approaches. If you are like many of my boot camp or triathlon friends, I have heard it's not "tough" enough for you and isn't a "workout." Think again. Yoga is life-changing. Give it a shot and watch how it impacts your mind, body, and soul. It can help you boost your immune system and manage chronic illness too. For years, yoga to me was a great way to sweat and in my mind "de-tox" and find peace, but now it's gone beyond that. Without yoga I couldn't manage the neuropathy damage that my chemo caused. Yoga is how I am able to function.

For years, I have to beg my hard-core weekend warriors who love intense workouts to please join me in a hot yoga class. Whether it was a friend or simply a doubter, I would invite friends and strangers to class and then interview them afterwards. The response was amazing: https://www.sciencedaily. com/releases/2018/05/180510101254.htm

Trinity College Institute of Neuroscience and the Global Brain Health Institute made this breath brain connection. It says, "The research shows for the first time that breathing—a key element of meditation and mindfulness practices—directly affects the levels of a natural chemical messenger in the brain called noradrenaline. This chemical messenger is released when we are challenged, curious, exercised, focused or emotionally aroused, and, if produced at the right levels, helps the brain grow new connections, like a brain fertilizer."

It goes on to say that the way we breathe directly affects the chemistry of our brains in a way that can enhance our attention and improve our brain health.

So, let's get started.

Breathe

There is a Zen proverb that says, "You should sit in meditation for twenty minutes a day, unless you are busy; then you should sit for an hour."

You should sit in meditation for twenty minutes a day, unless you are busy; then you should sit an hour.

Dr. Sukhraj Dhillon

No meditation, no life.
Know meditation, know life

Dr. Sukhraj Dhillon

It is powerful. It speaks to me and if you are going non-stop like I did and living life burning the candle at both ends, then this should speak to you as well. If you are so busy that you can't even stop for twenty minutes then you likely need an entire hour each day to meditate, and to withdraw from your problems—to reflect, BREATHE and find peace within your soul. Then, you might need to rethink how busy your life is and where you can make some changes. Trust me, I didn't even have twenty minutes to meditate, I wasn't about to make time for it, and guess what? I had an entire year to do it when I sat in that hospital.

Find time to pause, or your life will find it for you.

Find time to BREATHE.

In Dr. Dhillon's book, *The Power of Breathing,* he gives a great analogy, one more thing to consider when I urge you to maintain the car and maintain your body. He says, "Poor breathing is to low energy as bad air filter is to low car performance." So, let's talk about breathing.

Yes . . . it is as easy as taking ten minutes a day to take deep breaths in and deep breaths out. If you go to yoga, you will work on this type of breathing often. One type of deep breathing is called *Pranayama,* which literally means "to extend the vital life force," or *prana,* is an incredibly rich practice made up of many breathing techniques I want you to take a deep breath now and try it.

Breathe in with me. Slowly, in through the nose, fill the lungs. 1-2-3-4. Hold it. . . (four to eight seconds) and breathe out with pursed lips. . . and breathe in for 1-2-3-4, Hold it and breathe out. AGAIN. When you do this, air will fill your lungs, your lower belly will rise. If you can start making a habit to just do ten breaths like this a day, you will feel the difference.

Do these types of exercises in yoga, guided imagery and mindfulness meditation are just a few ways to counteract your stress response.

Deep breathing increases the supply of oxygen to your brain and stimulates the parasympathetic nervous system, which promotes a state of calmness.

The study looked at what's called natural killer (NK) cells (a type of cell critical to the body's immune system) and found that controlled rhythmic *breathing* increased NK cells over a three to six-month period. It's not a quick fix, but it's a positive step in the right direction.

https://pubmed.ncbi.nlm.nih.gov/16387692/

Below are some additional methods to lowering stress both during cancer treatment and during healthy times, leading to relaxation, feeling better, comfort.

- *Cancer hats*

  Fancy is great, but I really suggest an all-cotton hat, especially for sleeping. My head was sweating then freezing all day and night! I rarely used the fancy hats, but used the cotton ones daily and sweated through so many each day

- *Medical massages*

  Get a medical massage approved & send someone! This person has to understand cancer and how to properly massage a patient with low platelets. The doctor must clear it, but it is so worth it. I just wanted to be held and touched so badly because of my pain and this made a huge difference with my pain and anxiety.

- *Reiki*
- *Lighted candles (battery-operated)*
- *Comforter (twin size for the hospital bed)*
- *Memory foam pillow*
- *Organic lotion*

  NO fragrance—NO perfume. Your skin gets raw. And sunscreen is a must too. Your skin gets thin. Chemo burns through your skin if you go outside, and that can cause a fever. I would walk with my IV pole outside the hospital for fresh air, but got burned and ended up very sick. I got scolded. It's tough being in the hospital with no way to buy these things. I sent my hubby on a rat race

- *Lip gloss*
- *Chapstick*
- *Picture collages* (for the wall, pillowcase, cards, etc.)

- *Artificial flower arrangements*

   THIS can brighten up a room! REAL flowers were not allowed on my unit, and while this may have changed, it's even better to have a beautiful vase of fun flowers to brighten the room day after day!

Acupuncture

Post bone marrow transplant, acupuncture has been part of my routine in recovery. While some Western doctors may not embrace the ancient practice, others encourage it and that is wonderful news. I find it very healing for my body.

Acupuncture, a 3000-year-old healing technique of traditional Chinese medicine, has been shown in studies to reduce and/or manage pain and stress and aid in overall well-being, from boosting your immune system to balancing hormones. It helped me lower my stress levels and boost my progesterone when everyone told me there was no way I would ever get pregnant. It worked when nothing else did. I defied the odds. I trust it to help me to do the same in this phase of my journey post-cancer. Acupuncture has been a part of my life for a long time. It's been successful for me as a complement to the Western medicine that I'm so grateful ultimately saved my life.

Spiritual

The Armor of God, whoever your God is. Get a relationship. Find your faith. Surround yourself with prayer warriors.

Now more than ever people are dealing with anxiety, loneliness, depression, and restlessness, but now we are being given an opportunity to spend some time to just be still. It is a time for re-centering, time for prayer, time for introspection, time for gratitude. Even though we are trying to keep our minds occupied, this is the time we can be still.

***

It took me an entire month in isolation at the hospital to realize that I needed to take time to slow down, give myself grace, talk to God, and reset my intentions. During COVID-19, fear and loneliness spread as fast as the virus. It's times like these when your spirituality can bring you strength to cope.

"The Lord will fight for you, you need only to be still." -- Exodus 14:14

Financial

A GoFundMe is not a plan, but it's the only reason we didn't lose our house. I may have prepared physically for the fight, but I had no idea how unprepared we were financially and legally. You might be finding this out the same thing after COVID-19.

Cesar and I both had great careers at the time of my diagnosis. We knew we were in for a physical fight, but had no idea how financially devastating it could be. We were in awe of how we struggled financially to fight cancer. The stress of the financial toxicity almost killed me with worry of how to pay our bills, and how we weren't going to get bad credit (we did), and how we were going to make it from one house payment to the next.

Add to that the fact that, under extreme stress and not of sound mind, this was not the time to make life or death legal decisions. I will never forget looking up at a Johns Hopkins staff member with a clipboard in his hands to go over these tough decisions. His face was so blurry, and his voice cracked as he looked at me and I appeared in such pain. He said, "Hi Mrs. Hernandez-Aldama, I'm here to help you with some important decisions. Do you have a will or advanced directive? How about guardianship for your mom to care for your son? And how about a DNR (do not resuscitate) order?"

"Uhhhh Wha. . . ? What?" I could barely sit up. "Excuse me?" I put my hands on my then-bald, cold, sweaty head and stuttered, "Uh, uh, uh, no. I don't have any of that. Can you help me?"

Whether you are a patient, a caregiver, or on the sidelines in quarantine, the financial toxicity of illness is devastating. Cancer patients deal with this struggle daily. I cannot encourage you enough to wave the flag, reach out to friends, and ask for help. We are all stronger together.

One health catastrophe is all that stands between most families and financial ruin. It's been years now since my leukemia went into remission, and we're still digging out from the wreckage. Even though we were lucky enough that a lot of my treatment was covered by health insurance through Cesar's plan, we were spending thousands of dollars out of pocket every month. The added costs piled up. There were copayments for everything—my hospital room, the chemo cocktail and dozens of prescriptions, the never-ending blood work (by an out-of-network provider), care from doctors and medical techs and skilled nurses, scans and lab cultures.

The big one was IV Tylenol. Never heard of it? Neither had I, and it costs $1,000 a pop. Insurance covered only the pill form. For a lot of my time in chemo, I could barely eat or swallow because of mucositis—miserably painful inflammation and ulcers in the digestive tract that are a barbaric side effect of the toxins. When mine was bad, I couldn't even drink through a straw. Everything—water, drugs, nutrients—had to come through my IV. Now remember, I wasn't taking the heavy-duty pain meds for the most part. Still, at times we had no choice.

TAKEAWAY

Money shouldn't come between us and survival. I was going to live at all costs. Sadly, with healthcare disparities, money plays a big one in patient outcomes.

Our travel costs, of course, were through the roof since my mom was keeping Gabriel in Atlanta. Even with the generous break Southwest Airlines gave us on last-minute booking, tickets back and forth for them to visit between treatment cycles ran around $1,500 (Cesar would round-trip it on both ends to help them fly). And Cesar flew down there every other weekend in an effort to keep connected to our son.

Another complicating factor was our recent move: Nearly everything belonging to Gabriel and me was still boxed away somewhere in our new, unlived-in house. We had to buy replacement clothes and toys for him in Georgia. Preschool and after-school care in Atlanta was a hefty bill, plus we helped out with my mom's grocery bill. And every month our mortgage and insurance payments came due—for a home we'd purchased based on the expectation of *two* incomes. Now that was a big mistake.

Add to all of that in Cesar's overnight parking at the hospital garage, the extra gas and tolls needed to shuttle back and forth between work, Hopkins and home, plus easily $40 a day for meals he ate out (the man had no time or place to cook). Healthy groceries and snacks for me rounded out our basic expenses. In the middle of everything, Cesar's car broke down and needed a $6,000 transmission repair. It was nuts. And that was before the massive bills we amassed during my bone marrow transplant.

At the beginning, before we redirected delivery of our bills, my husband would collect whatever piled up in the mailbox at our house in Virginia and hand me the stack. I would sit on my bed with my laptop, prioritize the bills, and pay what I could online. Thank God for online bill pay! That's right, staring death in the face and hooked to an IV chemo drip, I was running our household finances. Doctors or nurses would come into my room to do a test, and I'd be on the phone begging some creditor to be flexible about our payments. It was exhausting, and it was distracting.

There was no patient navigator to suggest, "Hey, you can call these companies and tell them you have a medical emergency and ask for some leniency." Nope. No guidance toward a financial crisis plan. This is what I hope ArmorUp for LIFE® can do one day for other patients. Financial fitness matters.

I knew what I needed to do. Delegate and ask for help. I wasn't going to make it if I didn't wave that white flag. Time to call up the pit crew. My friend Alyce jumped in with both feet. "Get over your pride," she said. "Let's just ask for help." We accepted her offer to do a GoFundMe campaign, to raise money for our expenses through social media.

Cesar and I were humiliated. We had never asked anyone to help us financially. We were the ones who'd always done the donating, whether it was to worthy organizations or people in need. But suddenly all the good karma we had put out into the world over our lifetimes came rushing back. I was never so glad that I'd put good into the world and helped others, because now so many people helped us. I am grateful to this day, and will always pay it forward.

My husband never got comfortable with the idea of accepting charity. Even though we were in desperate shape and could have lost our home, he would tell people we were good and turn their offers away. It's just his nature.

Of course, a GoFundMe money-raising campaign is not supposed to be a financial plan. But it was what we wound up with. Cesar and I were still young, fairly well-situated with good incomes, and focused on our careers. We hadn't set aside savings properly—not because of lavish lifestyles, but because we'd been living apart in two distant households and often aiding other family members. We figured it would be decades before we needed to worry about having a financial cushion. Now we were paying the price.

We have all heard financial planners say everyone should have six months of living expenses saved up for emergency situations, and it sounds wise. Sadly, no one ever thinks those experts are talking about them. We're lucky. Cesar's salary and the GoFundMe account kept us afloat. But the perfect credit ratings from our earlier lives have unraveled. No credit bureau adds the disclaimer BUT SHE BATTLED LEUKEMIA!! when they downgrade your status.

Diet, exercise, lifestyle, spiritual and financial fitness all play a crucial role in your overall well-being.

Start building your pit crew today.

CHAPTER 7

Present Well to All Your Medical Team

Spend any time at a hospital unit and no doubt you will hear the phrase as doctors make their rounds, "How does the patient present?" or "Patient presents with these symptoms. . . x, y, and z." Basically, it means when they assessed you, how did they find you? What current symptoms you are exhibiting, physically and mentally? What are you diagnosed with and what underlying conditions, or baggage, do you bring to the table?

All of these answers will play a role in your course of treatment and how aggressively your medical team thinks you can be treated based on what you can physically handle. We hear this time and time again with COVID-19. Do you have respiratory issues? Diabetes, or other illnesses that will complicate your course of treatment? How far can they physically push your limits without killing you while trying to save you?

I remember the day I checked into Johns Hopkins. I was in complete denial even as they sent me down on a stretcher to radiology to have my Hickman inserted into my chest, allowing nurses to send the chemo directly into my heart and through my veins. At the time, I had still refused to put a gown on for fear that the gown itself would dash my hope. I was in my usual athletic gear. While I did look exhausted, I looked fit, apart from the symptom of "swollen belly".

The radiology team said, "Wait? You're the patient? You have leukemia? You don't look sick."

I was proud at that moment that I didn't *look* sick. It also fed into my denial of the actual seriousness of my illness. I smiled through tears and said, "Yep. I have leukemia. My son was just taken away from me and they tell me I will be here for a year."

Mentally I was cracking, but physically I "presented" well. I was assessed by the world-class medical team and was told, "There are not enough studies based on your mutation for AML and on patients of Hispanic background, but what we can tell you is, you are FIT (note: I had just completed a triathlon). From a cardiovascular standpoint your heart is in excellent condition. Your blood pressure is perfect. You have no underlying medical conditions. We believe you can handle the strongest dose of chemo. It won't be easy, but we feel strongly that, given how you 'present,' we will be able to push your limits and max out your doses. It may take a year, but this will give you the best possible chance of survival."

I was *one* of the lucky ones.

Others, including a woman and her husband I met late one evening, couldn't tell the same story. Her husband was sobbing in the halls and talked to me as I walked my laps. He told me they tried to check her into the leukemia unit but instead they had to send her to cardiology. He cried to me. He felt hopeless. He said, "She can't even check in. They told me she must first get her heart strong enough before they can treat her. The chemo is so toxic. She needs a strong heart." The chemo runs straight through the heart. Again, it was the same message of "we can't kill you trying to save you."

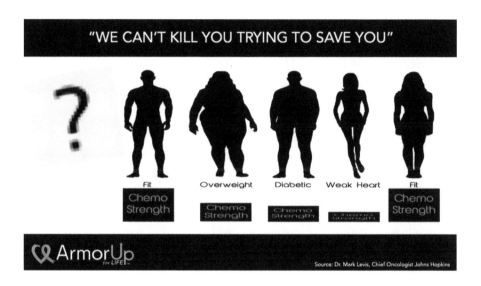

Once I learned that, it did help me feel a sense of control that I had a role in my success. OMG, who would want to half-fight for his or her life and get a watered-down dose? I would imagine, no one! But I wonder about others who weren't so ready (by their own lack of preparedness). Do you think they would do things differently if they knew how they prepared their bodies for this moment was determining their dose of treatment? I felt like I needed to share this message with the world. I wanted to shout it from the mountaintop.

So, I ask you to take a moment and do some self-reflection and assessment. How would you "present" if you face an illness like cancer, COVID, or some other sickness? Would you get the big aggressive bag of chemo, or would you need a watered-down version because you showed up with too much medical baggage?

How a patient *presents* matters. And while I am actively advocating for hospitals to open PREhab clinics to help you, the patient, really get prepared before a surgery or treatment ahead, your PREhab needs to start *today* long before any illness arrives. You don't need to wait for an illness.

It's a similar story for COVID-19. We can do all the social distancing and quarantine we want, but there is still a chance you might get it. The thought of contracting a virus that has killed so many is terrifying, but wouldn't you feel better knowing that IF it happens, you are going to go through it stronger than ever before? Would that give you a sense of grit and determination to push and have a will to survive? It is that very mindset that kept me alive during my fight.

I know it's not a guarantee, but if you have a 25 or 50 percent chance of survival, wouldn't you want ALL 25 or ALL 50 percent, not a percent less?

PRESENT well to your medical team. It will be the best PRESENT to yourself.

My favorite quote is one that Steve Jobs, the co-founder and CEO of Apple, gave on his deathbed, and boy does it ring true to all of us. It is something I have said time and time again through the battle cry of my ArmorUp for LIFE® movement and that the true meaning of wealth in your life is your health. He said, "What is the most expensive bed in the world? —Sick Bed. You can employ someone to drive your car for you, make money for you, but you cannot have someone to bear the sickness for you.

Material things lost can be found. But there is one thing that can never be found when it is lost — Life."

Yes, you cannot pay anyone to carry the disease for you. Whatever the disease or illness may be, you will be the one fighting. You can't pay someone else.

Present well.

CHAPTER 8

Prevail

You prepared, you presented well to your medical team, and now you have PREVAILED! Congratulations! This is no easy feat. It definitely took mind over matter and finding the courage and strength to overcome the adversity. If it's not cancer, it could be something else you overcame, but if you have gone through illness or adversity of any kind, you know this feeling. There is no greater feeling than overcoming the odds and winning. To those who have to do it over and over again (me!), find strength in adversity. We have to jump hurdles and navigate roadblocks. Sometimes I feel like I'm jumping over landmines. Stamina is needed to stand through the storm. We need the tenacity, and a "don't take no for an answer" attitude, in order to triumph.

If you are reading this and you haven't faced major obstacles yet, know that at some point in your life, you probably will. But rest assured, the sense of control you will crave will be satisfied by knowing you were prepared. Trust me.

The good news is, after preparing and presenting well, you have positioned yourself for success and it worked. It's clear there are no overnight remedies to achieve prosperity to overcome, but rather a combination of elements overtime. But you won! Yay! I'm so happy for you. But warning. . . it doesn't mean you let your guard down. Yes, breathe a sigh of relief, celebrate, and then get back to preparing. I know. I know. I'm relentless. Trust me, you will thank me. I will share why later in the book. Another challenge might be waiting in the wings, but this time you know you are prepared. Once you prevail, go back and repeat the cycle. Start preparing again. Make it a lifestyle. A cycle of success. A mantra.

Here's why. Years after I coined the term ArmorUp for LIFE® and launched the 3P's to surviving illness, we are finally making headway. Here is a quote that validates my message and should speak volumes to continuing the cycle of success through the 3P's. It is a statement from the Chair of the Clinical Oncology Society of Australia. He said, "If we could turn the benefits of exercise into a pill it would be demanded by patients, prescribed by every cancer specialist, and subsidized by government—it would be seen as a major breakthrough in cancer treatment."

He added another message to cancer patients, a message which is powerful and reiterates my message. "Withdrawing from exercise after diagnosis or while undergoing treatment actively harms cancer patients' chances of survival."

Now What?

For cancer patients, once we prevail, we often say, now what?

"Go out and start living!" That's what everyone tells us. That's what, in our hearts, we want to do.

But there's no clear easy path to surviving illness.

It is hard to fight cancer, but it's also hard to survive it. In fact, it is *very* stressful to survive. Yes, I said it. Sounds crazy to put it this way, but survivors will understand me when I say it. I went from fighting for my life to at times wanting to take my own life. The emotional and mental struggle is real. Therapy is what helps me cope with my unresolved trauma.

You have spent how many months or years having a medical team tell you in a very gray middle-of-the road fashion, "we will do the best we can", and "we will fight this aggressively." They would never commit to a resounding "Yes" or a definite "No" when I asked if I would survive and see my son again. Just gray. Nothing black or white. The ambiguity of it all drove me nuts. After years in TV and as a news anchor and reporter, I was used to yes or no answers. You either did it or you didn't, right? This whole "maybe" part leads to stress, anxiety, and depression.

You can tell us to go live life but secretly there is a fear of the other shoe dropping. After all, depending on the type of drugs, chemo and/or radiation can play a role in our "new normal." I HATE that phrase. Many of us are left with an array of problems, including neuropathy-like burning feet, heart disease from the chemo, cognitive issues that impact our thinking and (even more traumatizing) secondary cancers. For example, the drugs and chemo put me at a very high risk of melanoma and the full-body radiation put me at risk of other cancers.

But while I suffer from PTSD (post-traumatic stress disorder) and unresolved trauma, and you might too, I also have experienced post-traumatic growth. This is what keeps me going. The growth is what inspires me. Prevailing and overcoming can have a transformational role in our personalities. Like the saying from a German philosopher goes, "What doesn't kill you makes you stronger." It certainly does. In fact, a study published by https://psycnet.apa.org/record/2010-21218-001 the American Psychological Association (APA) confirmed that adverse experiences can in fact foster resilience, that people (we survivors) who have gone through so much are less affected by other adverse events. Basically, we have a much different perspective than those who haven't gone through what we have had to overcome.

Surviving has certainly helped me find meaning and purpose in my life. There is thought behind every single thing I do and every single decision I make. I often find myself going overboard making memories because I worry if the other shoe will drop. The "what if" monster always rears its ugly head.

You came out of this stronger. Pull strength from your resilience. You will find even more purpose in everything. You will see life through a much different lens. You have a new chance at life, so what are you going to do with it? How are you going to pay it forward? Who can you help? What changes will you make in your own life? What toxic relationships will you get rid of? This is a time of self-reflection to look back on your past and let it reshape and define how differently you will move forward to your new norm.

But please know this—suffering with the unresolved trauma and also having post-traumatic growth can both exist. It does for me. Do know it is okay to be angry. It is okay to feel lost. It is okay to be depressed. It is okay to feel frustrated with the process of putting the pieces back together and moving forward. I've been there. Many days I am still there. I know the drill.

I continue to eat clean (no gluten, no dairy, no sugar, no caffeine) and exercise, but now I have added in SLEEP. After all the doctors shared so much about the impact of sleep deprivation on the body, I'm terrified of NOT sleeping. I now know the statistics and the impact it can make on my body. I know that when you don't sleep you don't restore cells. I know it can deplete the bone marrow which is the source of the very cancer I faced. I know where it can land me. . . right back in the cancer ward. Some studies have shown *lack of sleep* appears to lower white *blood cell count,* which suggests a compromised immune system. What happens when you are compromised? You are more susceptible to illnesses when you are sleep-deprived.

This is the bottom line. Once you prevail, you need another strategy and pit crew to keep on living and to get back up.

Ask for the help you need. Wave that flag.

We are all here to support you.

And if you fight another fight, we will be here again. Remember, you prepared.

There is a saying by Confucius that nails it on the head: "The man (woman) who moves a mountain begins by carrying away small stones." And it's much easier to get started with small stones when we don't realize how big the mountain really is.

Start moving the small stones. Rejoice in your victory. Embrace life. Make Memories. Take your vacations. Spread kindness. Get prepared. Get prepared over and over and over again. Present well again and you will once again be positioned to PREVAIL.

CHAPTER 9

The Fight of My Life

Shared Decision-Making

There is a lot of talk (and fascination) in the medical community about how much shared decision-making there is during a cancer diagnosis, or any other for that matter. Shared decision-making is where the patient and physician both take an active role in the decision-making process to determine the best course of treatment and care. For me, there were different levels of shared decision-making depending on what part of the journey/process I was in. For the most part, it wasn't shared at all.

At the time of diagnosis, there was no shared decision-making. I had no say or voice except that I knew I was going to Johns Hopkins and I wasn't going back to where I was misdiagnosed ever again. After that, when it came to treatment options and if I was going to harvest my eggs for another baby to use in the future, I had no voice. Earlier in the book, I shared how I wanted to freeze my eggs and wait fourteen days before chemo started. I asked to see a fertility specialist. They did send someone from within Johns Hopkins to come talk to me, but the doctors advised against it and insisted my life was on the line and fourteen days could mean life or death for me. My husband said no and that was the end of the story. While I understand I wasn't of sound mind to make that decision. I wanted to have a second baby no matter what, so that decision, or lack of it, left me feeling like a lunatic. Despite my heartache and sadness, this was one time I look back and I know they made the right decision for me. But take note, nothing was shared.

Throughout my treatment, nothing was really shared.

When I decided to refuse all pain meds so I could be fully present, ArmorUp for LIFE®, and walk each day and not be a foggy version of myself, I made that decision. I was told repeatedly to not be so hard on myself but I didn't like the way they made me feel so I refused them.

When I enrolled in clinical trials, I turned to Dr. Levis and his expertise to make both decisions. I had no idea what the researchers were talking about and didn't know what was best for me and my survival, so I relied on Dr. Levis to make the call. When I pulled myself out of the trial, it was because I was advised it was too risky to stay in the trial and be randomized.

I knew I was blessed with such an incredibly brilliant oncologist, so I relied heavily on his expertise and held onto his every word. While I did push back often and question the process and decisions made, I trusted Dr. Levis because he was world-renowned and had the experience to back him.

I do worry about those at oncology centers where treatment isn't customized and there aren't teams of doctors, but rather one doctor and there is no shared decision-making. While Dr. Levis was my primary doctor, a team of doctors always "rounded" on my case. That means they discussed it as a team and each doctor weighed in with his or her insight as to the best way to move forward.

Now, let's take you to "Cycle One" of four long cycles of chemo.

End of Cycle One

Week by week, the chemo did its dirty work and my blood cell counts kept dropping. They were finally at zero. It's as if my body was a car, and the toxic drugs had stripped it down to just a shell. Now it was time to build me back up and let my engines roar! As soon as my white blood cells, red blood cells, and platelets reached safe levels, I could go home to Virginia for a week and a half. Cesar would fly to Atlanta, pick up my mom and Gabriel, and bring them back to visit me. That process could take anywhere from twenty-eight to forty-five days, depending on how long the rebound actually took.

I waited impatiently as my engine started to sputter and slowly produce cells. How long it takes to start over is different for everyone—it depends on how healthy you were to start with, on how much chemo you have received, and how your body processes it. The toxic effects compound themselves over time. Some patients never go back to generating cells, and they die. For each treatment cycle I received, my recovery took more time.

I walked and walked and walked to build my strength. Each day my blood counts rose closer to the target range where they could sustain me. At morning rounds, my medical team would tell me, "You are close. Maybe tomorrow you can go home." But tomorrow often turned into days or maybe even another week as my heart ached for Gabriel. This was one area I could not control and it frustrated me.

I was so excited to get out of there, but also scared of what I'd find. On social media I kept posting my fear that Gabriel would have forgotten me. Everyone assured me, "a child never forgets his mommy. You breastfed him for twenty months. He *will* remember you." They made me think I was crazy.

In the Hollywood-style reunion I pictured, I would joyfully lift Gabriel in the air and swing him around. We'd giggle. I would play that scene over and over in my head.

Break #1

At last, the day came. Cesar flew to Atlanta, brought Gabriel and my mom back on the plane, and drove them to the hospital. They called me from the first floor, since children weren't allowed upstairs. I took the elevator down, wearing my hat to cover my still-bald head. Across the lobby I saw Cesar—and there was Gabriel. I ran to my child, yelling, "Gabriel, Gabriel, Mommy is back. I love you."

The boy looked at me like a deer caught in headlights, then ran to Cesar to hide behind his leg. He walked past me like we had never met. It was one of the most painful moments of my entire motherhood. My son ran *from* me. How could this be? After forty-five days apart he didn't recognize me, and this was only phase one of a long year of separation ahead. Did he no longer need me? My heart was broken.

I was so angry. Where was the mental health help? Where was the patient navigator at this world-class institution to help me cope? The one psychologist I got to see, only after begging to see her, saw me for fifteen minutes, tops. First, she questioned why I couldn't see Gabriel. That pissed me off. Why was I explaining my treatment and my blood counts to her? Should she not know this? Adding insult to injury, during her whopping fifteen minutes, she assured me my son wouldn't forget me. He did.

I needed help. I didn't have it. Why was equal value not placed on mental health as much as physical health? I was a whole person facing real-life problems while fighting for my life. Making matters worse, there was no reintegration program like the military offers veterans for these brief three to five-day visits I might get every few months in the year ahead. No one to help the transition. The move. The unpacking. I just went from chemo running through my veins one day to unpacking a house the next. That time should have been spent with re-establishing a bond with my son.

Our house in Northern Virginia was a mess. Moving boxes were still everywhere. And I couldn't be around dust or germs. My mom was freaking out. It was so *stressful*. At the very first chance I could, I laid on the couch with Gabriel and stared into his eyes, hoping he would look back into mine instead of past them. His look was empty, like a stranger had picked him up and tried talking to him. Not the look a child who breastfed for twenty-two months might give his mom. There was no twinkle. No sparkle. Just a blank stare. I had lost him. Not physically but emotionally. The bond. Our connection was gone. I just cried. Tears rolled down my face as he looked through me, past me; strangely, he would use his little fingers to dry my tears.

We started opening boxes, looking for toys Gabriel could play with or clothes he could wear. In one, Gabriel discovered a hairbrush and picked it up. He toddled over to me, sat in my lap, and said, "Brush. Brush?" What happened next, I will never forget. He tugged my hat off, got a confused look on his face, then started crying and wouldn't stop. I had never let him see me bald. Who was I? Who was this woman staring into his eyes? I was a stranger to my son. I was a stranger to myself.

We passed those few days together. We snuggled day and night, and I tried to enjoy each moment. Because of my infection susceptibility, we couldn't leave the house. But I didn't want to see or talk to anyone else anyway—even if we had known people in our new community. I just wanted to hold my son.

On the last day we did risk leaving the house just once—to attend the circus. Yes, a circus. My life felt like one. It was risky with my immune system, but I was desperate to make memories. I kept saying, "One more memory. One more memory," just in case I died. I wanted one more story for Gabriel to hold in his heart. Friends had given us tickets to view the show from a suite, away from everyone. Gabriel looked into my eyes and said, "Mama, love you," and giggled. It was worth every second. It was a magical memory.

I was *finally* reconnected with my son. I wasn't sure he really understood who I was but we snuggled and I started to see him look at me differently. Sadly, as soon as I felt any progress made, I had to tell him goodbye *again*. I had to return to the hospital for the next cycle of treatment.

I held Gabriel in my arms and kissed him, once again not knowing if I would ever see him again. This time he was four months older, and he looked so confused. I was sobbing hysterically. "Mommy loves you," I choked in a whisper. "Mommy is walking for you and doing all I can. Please know I love you with all my heart. I'm going to the store. I'll be back as soon as I can."

He screamed, "Mommy! Mommy!" with his arm reached toward me.

This wasn't like a girl's beach trip that I could cancel out of guilt. This was life or death. I quickly handed him to my mom, who had her own tears rolling down her face. She couldn't give in to worries about her own daughter while she stepped in to parent her grandson.

I still have flashbacks of those horrible goodbyes. But I put faith over fear, believing God had bigger plans for me. I wasn't done with my fight. Cesar and I drove away toward Johns Hopkins. We said nothing. We were numb. I gazed out the window. I was speechless. What the hell was happening? How did I deserve this?

Back for Round Two

As we headed back to the hospital, I was angry and in tears. A deep part of me wanted to turn around right then and there, take the short-term reward and stay with Gabriel. And yet, I wasn't ready to die, I kept telling myself throughout the entire drive. Looking at the big picture, I gambled it was worth our separation and the mortal risk of chemo if it meant I could spend a lifetime watching my boy grow up. *Faith over fear.* I had to put it into action.

When we got to Johns Hopkins, I rolled in with my huge suitcase. I always received stares when I rolled up with that suitcase. It wasn't my first rodeo. I was prepared with everything I might need. Vitamix, hand weights, fitness gear, computer, customized pic collage blankets to pin to the wall, pictures to post everywhere, nutrient-dense snacks like homemade granola, protein power, battery-operated candles, my rosary beads, holy water, sneakers, slippers, bras for jogging with no wires for easy CT scanning, and more. I was ready to step back in that ring like a champ. *No one* comes between a mother and her child—not even fucking cancer!

I got my new room assignment and began setting up my life for the next who-knew-how-many weeks . . . months. I hung photo collages of Gabriel and Cesar all over the walls, stacked my walking pants and tops, sneakers, underwear, tank tops and more. I fluffed my treasured comforter atop the bed, and set out battery-operated candles to soften the atmosphere.

A nurse brought me my new calendar with dates for chemo and target blood-count rates along the way. My treatment cycle would be more of the same: kill cells, grow healthier cells to restart body, then (after a break) — bam! — turn around and do it again. And again. Each of the four cycles I endured was longer than the last.

There were chemo days, days for other drugs, notes for what my blood counts should be at different stages. Blank spaces were left to record my progress. This was my road map for Cycle 2. But it didn't point to how the journey would end.

Patient Deaths

I wanted a guarantee that I would survive. People were dying all around me. Even in my first stay for treatment at the hospital,

I'd lost friends on my hall. It was devastating. It was surreal. One day you see them. The next day you don't. Just like that. The name plate was removed from the door and a new name went up for the next one to step into the ring and attempt to beat the odds. It felt like a revolving door. I was baffled.

When I cried to Dr. Levis about so much loss around me and how it was hard to focus on living when everyone was dying, he responded with, "Don't make friends."

What? You might think that's a bit bold or harsh, but that's Dr. Levis for you. Take him or leave him. He knows his work and doesn't mince words. He's transparent. He's real. He is a world-renowned oncologist but he had to double as a therapist. I always felt bad that this brilliant man whose expertise was in leukemia had to also do the work of a "therapist." I used to worry about his workload. He was like this superhero. He was and is brilliant and as real as it gets. He always broke things down in layman's terms for me and others.

But how could we not make friends? These patients became our only family. We formed our own community. We relied on each other. We took care of one another. Their caregivers took care of me when Cesar worked. To cope, you needed a community. To potentially get out of there alive, you needed to form your own village.

But we patients knew the drill. An announcement would come over the P.A. telling us: "Return to your rooms." In other instances, the nurses would tell us to go back to our rooms. Then the chaplain would show up, and the shrieks of loved ones echoed through my door. Crying family members filled the halls—we could tell who it was by where they gathered and who wasn't out walking the next day.

And just like that, a friend was gone. Maybe the same friend I walked with the day before. They were people I depended on in my survival community. People who had dreams just like mine, to go home to their kids. Together we'd share victories and challenges from our earlier lives, but most of all regrets about not spending enough time with loved ones. We talked about focusing too much on accumulating money we couldn't take with us, about missing the warning signs our bodies had sent.

That was enough to make me realize *I needed to hedge my bets.*

The losses and devastation surrounding me and all patients painted a clear picture of yet another example of the lack of psycho-oncology and support for patients. Another area where so much work needs to be done.

Clinical Trials

Pomalidomide and sleep.

Drug-trial researchers were constantly visiting our floor looking to recruit patients for studies. And after all, we [cancer/leukemia] patients were a captive audience, fish in a barrel. "Would you enroll to help advance the cause of medicine?" they'd ask. At the time, there had been no advancements for forty years, so yes, we needed some to fast-track treatments.

Enrollment for drug trials is at a low 5 percent. That number always baffled me. It still does. Why? They (researchers) desperately wanted us. We desperately wanted to be a match for them, but no one could really speak our language. I found it disappointing that there was (and is) a big disconnect. It was beyond frustrating.

First, there is the mistrust, especially among communities of color. The "what are you doing with my research?" That is the unknown that will remain a big challenge for the research community, both with patients and with those minorities like myself. But I didn't see an effort to make me feel a connection or bond with the researcher either. There is more work to be done. Also creating a barrier is the lack of information and the delivery of this so-called knowledge.

I really, really wanted to sign up. Those on my unit did too. We were all desperate to be part of a trial. We desperately wanted to feel like there was hope. Somewhere. Anywhere. Sign me up! We would each shuffle through the halls and compare and almost gossip who was being considered for which study. We also agreed the process was overwhelming and confusing. We had so many questions, and the researchers often didn't have the answers or would look at us like unsuspecting deer caught in headlights. For starters, I kept saying, we can't *READ* the fine print if we can't *SEE* it. The chemo often affected our vision and it certainly did mine! I belonged to the 6 percent who had the displeasure of getting chemo burn in my eyes.

The reporter in me wanted to do a story on this enrollment process to advocate for a better system so we could boost participation and, eventually, survival rates. While I truly admire these professionals' dedication to the cause, the current strategy wasn't working. The whole process needed help. It needed an update. A complete overhaul. A consistent message. The timing and stoic monotone pitch with confusing paperwork set the tone.

Here's what I wanted to say. "Thank you! We need you. We love you. You are the brilliant researchers who might save me, but I'm lost. You aren't speaking my language. I get it, you are not a spunky sales team, but you are selling something—research—and your job is to convince me why I should sign up. Why I should take the risk? Why might this save my life? Why do I need you?

"I can understand what you are trying to tell me. You show up unannounced. Usually during the time that I am alone without my husband to help me interpret what exactly this trial means to my overall survival. I have just finished throwing up. I'm drenched in sweat, taking dozens of medications. Every five seconds I have diarrhea, and the room is spinning. I'm depressed, busy arguing with my insurance about what isn't covered (IV Tylenol), worried I'm going to die and, I have no idea what you are talking about. I can't read the fine print because my vision is so blurry. Heck, I can't even see the fine print. Is there a video I can watch to explain this to me before you walk in so I can be prepared?

"You showing up unannounced and expecting answers is like me calling you into a meeting without warning, not passing out an agenda, and asking for you to make a decision on a project I just presented (mumbled) to you for five minutes. Can you just draw a line on a piece of paper with the pros and cons to this trial? I mean really personalize this for me. All I really need to know is if I'm going to die—plain and simple.

"Wait—you need to know NOW? Can my doctor help me decide? Wait, I have to throw up again! OMG . . . okay . . . Will I live to see my son again? If so, where do I sign? Will I see him for just a few more years at least? Will I watch him grow up? Will I ever get to work again? If I sign up, can you guarantee to me that I will live? Will I just be broken? How long can I think about it? When will you come back? You don't know? Oh no . . . my husband isn't here to help me decide. Okay. I'll just ask my oncologist what is best. I'm too confused."

Maybe it was because I was overwhelmed and mostly alone, with too many other things to process there in the cancer ward. Or maybe the researchers needed to convey the message in a more conversational way. Coming from a news background I see everything in video. I would always ask, why is there not a preview video given to patients to set the stage prior to the researcher coming into our room? Make a video that says, "Hi! I'm so sorry you are going through tough times. I want you to know I understand what you are going through. I was you a few years ago. I know you have a lot of questions. But in the coming days/weeks a researcher will be coming to your room to discuss a study we feel you might be a great candidate for. We wanted to give you some information in advance so you and your caregiver could discuss it."

Wow! Wouldn't that be nice?

Now let's talk patient outcomes. I would always ask: "What will it do for me, or to me? And if I agree to try it, will it also increase my chances of dying?" I posed so many questions, and usually I didn't get answers. So, I would call Dr. Levis, my lead oncologist, and say, "What the hell is this drug they said I qualify for? What do you think? Can you put this into terms I can understand?

Dr. Levis is the most amazing human being on this planet. He would sit with me and explain every detail, in lay terms, describing what the trial drug was supposed to do. He might make an analogy to a queen bee and her hive, or a soldier in an army. Whatever the question, he had a simple, everyday comparison.

Forgive me when I say this, but that's not the norm for brilliant people. In my experience, when I was a TV reporter going to interview someone seriously brainy, it usually produced short, boring sound bites that I would have to chop up to make any use of. They had incredible messages and purposes but usually couldn't convey them in lay terms. In TV, finding brilliance *and* an accessible personality in the same package was tough. Dr. Levis was both and then some. He still is.

But with the invaluable input from Dr. Levis, I agreed to a couple of trials—one for a drug called Pomalidomide. I took it on top of that second round of chemo, even though I couldn't be sure what its consequences would be. To this day, I have no idea what the researcher told me. But I do know Dr. Levis thought it was a good idea. But I will never forget the side effects, like pouring sweat. I mean drenched from sweat. Sleeping was impossible. I did need sleep. We know sleep heals the body and allows it to restore cells. But, as I've described earlier in the chapter, sleeping in the hospital is not easy—and you won't be doing much of it at all if you're taking Pomalidomide. I still don't know if it saved my life, but the bottom line is: I signed up strictly because Dr. Levis thought it would be a good idea. It had nothing to do with what the researcher said.

It caused so many crazy side effects, on top of the long list caused by the chemo itself and my other treatments. But the sweating was unreal. I would wake up drenched several times during the night, but freezing and shivering from the wet sheets. Rita, one of the amazing nurses usually assigned to me, was the one always stuck with changing my sweat-drenched sheets countless times each night. It got so bad that she would stack nine sets of sheets in my room at the start of her shift. She never left my side. At least, it never felt that way. She was one of those amazing nurses that could be juggling six patients and make you feel like you were her only one.

If it wasn't sweat waking me up, it was a kinked catheter and the *beep, beep, beep* of the machine waking me up or nurses for medications throughout the night. Benadryl to keep me from breaking out in hives, for transfusions of platelets or red cells—followed by another blood draw later to see whether that worked.

Social/Emotional

I was exhausted. Being exhausted only messed with my already-fragile mental health.

I was beyond *stressed:* pulled from my child, facing every likelihood of death, traumatized by pain, and worried sick about money and what was happening to my family. And I was *depressed:* still reeling emotionally from being denied a second pregnancy, far from the friends, colleagues, and thousands of viewers who could support me, hopeless and confused about how a health-and-fitness guru like me could wind up with leukemia. I had gone from working hard to control everything in my life to feeling like I had no control at all.

Hormone/Weight

Then they messed with my hormones! That is an understatement. Because my platelets were dropping, I couldn't even have my period. If I bled, I would bleed to death.

But my body was going nuts. It had recently been primed for a pregnancy. So, after I'd been covered with hormone patches and received weeks of fertility shots to have the second baby that never would be, my doctors prescribed four—*yes, four*—different kinds of birth control. They wanted to make absolutely sure I wouldn't menstruate.

I got even crazier. I was losing it. I worried aloud that these life-saving precautions would make me fat, and then I would never be able to go back to an on-air career in TV. My doctors would look at me like I was out to lunch. "Your weight and your appearance should be the *last* thing you think about. You may very well die. Don't you get this?" And despite my own mortal fears, I would answer, "Listen, if I am going to go through all this shit to fight cancer, at least my ass can get smaller in the process! I can go back looking even better. I can't go back looking worse or my career will be over." Crazy, I know. I didn't know if I was going to live, but if I did, I wasn't sure how I was going to pay my bills and all the debt from fighting cancer.

And after twenty years in TV—having nearly every news director tell me to monitor my appearance and hint that I shouldn't gain a pound, even when I was rocking a Size 6 or 8—you develop a fear of putting on weight. I was told a million times every trick to look thinner. "Wear only V-necks to elongate your neckline. Don't wear double-breasted; it will make you look bigger. Have the camera held above you so you are looking up and can look thinner." I heard these over and over and over again.

Even talent agents would counsel, "You can report the best investigative story, but if you look like a mess, nobody will listen. They'll be tweeting about how you look."

That's the truth!

Bottom line, my doctors stopped my period for good. They threw me into menopause overnight. In one damn day, I lost any semblance of fertility, any dream of completing my family. Good luck with me keeping a positive outlook. When women complain about cramps and periods, I want to say, "I wish I had that problem."

Another day. Another loss. Another rip at my identity.

Mental Health

The lack of mental health care was the number-one void in my treatment, no question.

Doctors at the clinic had rallied immediately to form an extensive team to defeat my cancer. But no one was assigned to help me—or my family—navigate the huge challenges my treatment brought us. They need to rally another psycho-oncology team to come through after the medical team leaves your room. When the military sends soldiers into battle, there are whole systems to help prepare them and their families to handle the separation, stress, and risk of death or loss. That's part of what lets fighters just fight. Why shouldn't it be the same for patients in a cancer ward? Why isn't it?

Family

But we had no patient navigator to step in and guide us through a cascade of crises.

No one offered to find a therapist in the Atlanta area who could help my overstressed mom and traumatized son deal with having their worlds suddenly turned upside down. Even now as I write this, my son (now age eight) still talks about how he worried and wondered if I would ever come back to get him. My heartbroken husband has since told me that Gabriel didn't even recognize his own father when Cesar came to retrieve him from Georgia for our first two visits.

Yet each time when I had to part from my son to go back into the hospital, Gabriel would scream, "Where are you going?

As I sobbed uncontrollably, all I could get out was, "to the store."

People told me our child was so young that he wouldn't remember all that, so I believed it. But Gabriel has needed years of therapy for post-traumatic stress disorder (PTSD), with nightmares about death and fears I might never come home. Early on, when things fell apart and it was clear my mom couldn't care for Gabriel all by herself, I was the one online looking for sitters and caregivers near Atlanta—while hooked up to a chemo drip!

I broke down, crying to my nurses, "I can't die; no one knows how to care for our son!"

And the bills. The financial toxicity! The money! You've heard what a financial train wreck a major illness can be for people in this country. Well, it's true. And we had just gone from two incomes to one. I'll write about that mess later in this chapter. But let's just say, *we weren't prepared.*

In order to survive, it was important for me to focus on staying calm and fighting strong. Instead, I was putting out fires, one after another. My family and I needed help. The hospital did have a very kind social worker, Jessie, who was on assignment on our unit from the military. But he was stretched so thin, busy on rounds among hundreds of patients. He could spend only limited time with me—(like five minutes) when I was lucky enough to get an appointment (patients had to do the requesting). It wasn't enough for me to cope. I needed one-on-one psychological counseling. And not just for five minutes, but a regular, standing appointment. I had so many questions!

I asked my oncologist Dr. Levis to have a hospital psychologist come see me. Not for five minutes, not just for one visit, but on an on-going basis. I needed help and all I kept asking was, why there wasn't equal valued placed on mental and physical health. I was a whole patient with real-life problems, and needed support for both.

The psychologist who came, while assigned to the leukemia unit, was somehow not familiar with the realities of leukemia treatment. She would always ask me why Gabriel couldn't visit me during chemo and there I was explaining what my oncologist had just told me, oddly schooling *her* on the whys of separation. Gabriel's germs were a lethal risk to someone whose immune system was destroyed. He could kill me if I saw him.

Eventually I realized that if I was going to be an equal partner in my own success, *I* was the one who had to fix this problem. I called Dr. Allison Chase, the clinical child psychologist in Austin I had often interviewed on the air for many of my health and wellness segments at Fox 7. When I heard her familiar voice I broke down, spilling out all my desperation. She counseled me from afar as best as she could—and kept on doing so through my treatment, at no charge. I have no idea what I would have done without her.

With nothing but time on my hands at the end of the day, in the hours before Cesar arrived, sometimes I would do stupid things out of self-pity. I tried *to convince myself that no one cared* or understood my pain. I would stay out walking and walking, just to see if anyone gave a shit enough to come looking for me. Not the nurses—I knew they cared, sharing love and compassionate support every day. I just felt so alone. Some of my friends were busy with families and careers, 500 miles away in Texas. Others couldn't face the gravity of my situation. And my entire family was so overwhelmed holding down the fort in my absence, no one had time to ask me how I was doing—they just looked to me for what to do next.

Would anyone call? I wanted calls, but then I was too tired to take them. I just wanted someone to hold my damn hand and say it was going to be okay, and *really know* that it would be okay. I worried so much, I knew I had to add more to my schedule to stay *focused* on my survival plan.

Dr. Allison suggested a helpful distraction: spending more time on the photo albums I was putting together online for Gabriel. The idea was that, in case I died, these hardcover books would help him remember me. It was therapeutic, and I started blocking out two hours a day for that project.

I cried as I wrote each entry. I didn't just upload a ton of pictures to print, I put my heart and soul into these albums. I wrote notes to Gabriel by each picture, each memory. Told him how much I loved him, how he was my world, my love and light, and described what kind of boy I wanted him to grow up to be: kind, respectful and compassionate.

Otherwise, crazy things would pop into my head: I would be devastated just by a Facebook post I saw, like one from a woman dying of cancer who asked someone to marry her husband. I was like, whoa! I can't even think like that. Then the wheels would spin and I would tell Cesar, "Please don't remarry if I die. Please don't replace me so easily, like I was nothing."

All I could imagine was some other woman raising my son, letting him eat crappy food from McDonalds and neglecting his physical fitness. I couldn't get it out of my head; other people tried to console me by saying things like, "my first wife had cancer." *Oh, okay, so how many are you on now? How fast did you just pick up and move on?* I couldn't comprehend it.

I begged my husband almost daily to wait, if I died, before he remarried. I would ask Cesar ridiculous questions. How fast would you get over me? Who would this woman be? I became obsessed. Keep in mind, my husband is the most loyal man you could meet! But I was also taking an anti-fungal drug called voriconazole that had hallucinogenic side effects. Everything set me off and frightened me.

And yet, as crappy as that year was, kindness and *angels popped up all around me.* I was angry that I had leukemia but awestruck by those who came to my aid. In my daily social media posts about my battle, I tried to be transparent about what was going on, but I also tried not to sound as crazy as I was becoming. Still, my friends could read between the lines. They knew they couldn't take away my cancer, but they could help remove the noise. They sent friends of friends who lived in the Baltimore area to come and visit me: *angels among us.*

One Austin viewer who had come to Hopkins for a nursing study program just showed up one day. Jenny brought banana bread and sat with me. After I told her how much I missed being held, she made a habit of sneaking in to give me a light foot massage. She gave me rosary beads.

Another Austinite in the Johns Hopkins nursing program, Susannah, had worked for the Bikram yoga studio where I practiced. She also stopped by, and later brought me a heavy twin comforter to keep me warm. That was the best gift ever! Thin hospital blankets don't do the job when you are sick with fevers and chills, and they certainly don't feel like home.

Jenny and Susannah became heroes to me. Busy with school, they'd still duck into my room between classes, leave a surprise, blow me a kiss, gently rub my feet (ahhh, that *touch* meant so much!), and be on their way in a blink.

I will never forget this type of *unexpected kindness*.

Estrangements/Abandonment

But while complete strangers became friends, some long-time friends became complete strangers. They just disappeared. I was baffled. I called a few and asked what the hell had happened. I cried, and they admitted they didn't know what to say. Others who pretty well vanished, I realized my life exhausted them. Trust me. It exhausted me, but this was no time to disappear.

But I remained in awe of those I had not spoken to in years who jumped to my aid and reconnected and came back into my life. It was a blessing to gain new angels as I was losing others who couldn't handle the reality of my possible mortality.

TAKEAWAY

"If you have a friend or loved one going through cancer, please don't abandon them. Please keep in touch with him or her even by a simple text that says, "Thinking of you," or say, "I don't have the right words for you. I know you are struggling and I want you to know I'm thinking of you.""

Transfusions & Donor Difficulty

There were angels I never got to meet.

As a newswoman, I had done countless live reports at blood banks to encourage building up the local blood supply. I always imagined this was largely to benefit victims of traffic accidents. But back then I had no idea the amount of donated blood that cancer patients need to survive. I also had no idea that getting the right blood to patients wasn't just a matter of matching them with donors according to Type A, B or O, and positive or negative. Shouldn't an O-donation serve an O-negative patient? *Voila?* Actually, no.

In the hospital, I quickly learned that people can reject even their same type of blood because of antibodies—the proteins produced to counteract substances the body recognizes as alien, including bacteria and viruses. At times after a transfusion, nurses would come to inform me, "you didn't get a bump in your numbers. Your body didn't accept the platelets. We are going to call Dr. Platelet to see if we can find another donor who is a better match."

Dr. Platelet was the name of the office in Johns Hopkins where they stored the supply of donated platelets. Apparently, over months of transfusions, I had built up so many antibodies from so many transfusions that my body started to reject some—even from donors with my same blood type.

And yet, my platelet counts were at a bare minimum!

Eventually, it came down to *one* source, *one* donor in the hospital's bank whose blood I wouldn't reject. And there came a day that my numbers were so low, the team at Dr. Platelet reached out to this donor and asked him to come back sooner than his regularly scheduled donation. He did! I wanted to call and thank him, but there were privacy rules. I wanted to give that man a hug and tell him how much I was grateful for him.

Wrap-up of Round 2: Treatment Traumas & Bag Burst

To this day I'm not the bravest person when it comes to medical procedures—I fear the worst and get anxious. But there's reason for that: I know from experience the things that can go wrong.

One early morning (4:00 AM) during a chemo dosing, alone in my room and half-asleep, I heard a noise and felt a huge, wet splash. The chemo bag had fallen off the IV stand and burst! It was all over me. I jumped out of bed screaming. I was attached to the bag through the Hickman running into my heart, so I couldn't disconnect it and run away. A nurse came running, full of apologies, and we attempted to scrub the toxic drug off my skin. Then the *hazardous-materials team* came and cleaned up the spill.

All I kept thinking was that this toxic chemical—that everyone else has to suit up in protective gowns and gloves just to carry into my room—has been running *through my veins* for months Yes, this toxic chemical that requires a HAZ-MAT team to clean it up is the very chemical that is going into my body. It made me wonder what was happening inside my body and what long-term effects it might have.

The burst bag incident was written up but never addressed once again.

My Stressful Hickman

My infected Hickman in my chest was the source of so much stress.

One of the many days of suffering that stuck out was the day my Hickman got infected. I had been running fevers every day. We knew my blood counts had been knocked down by the chemo and that I had no immunity. But they couldn't find the source of the infection, and I got sicker and sicker. Ibuprofen was out of the question to bring my temperature down because it would thin out my blood. I was never allowed to have it. Tylenol was rarely allowed because, while it would lower the fever, it would also mask any infection that was threatening your life.

I was suffering. I was going downhill. Yet I made myself walk because I feared pneumonia. I was terrified to lay down. I was already using a breathing machine, and it was still hard to breathe. My long walks were replaced with shuffles and meant just putting one foot in front of the other. I was terrified. I was throwing up, I had shingles, I could barely move.

That night I continued to get worse. It was Sunday night and Cesar was supposed to go home to Virginia to get clothes for the week and have one solid night's sleep. So much for that idea. The nurses called Cesar to come back to the hospital immediately to be with me. It was so scary. I remember the nurse asking where Cesar was and suggesting he come back. I knew that didn't sound good. I knew what that meant. I worried I would be next, yet I felt bad bothering Cesar on his only night of rest. He grabbed clothes and was back at the hospital in less than ninety minutes. . . the amount of time to drive from our Virginia home to Johns Hopkins in Baltimore.

After days of trying to isolate the source of the problem, my doctors decided they needed to pull the Hickman out of my chest—by brute force. Holy shit! Back when they installed the catheter to feed drugs into my heart, I was under general anesthesia. But that wasn't an option. Now they were going to just one, two, three rip it out of my chest?

I was scared of dying and desperate for answers, so I agreed. What choice would I have? My best friend of twenty years, Natali Ceniza flew to be with me. She had hired me at CNN many years ago. She knew my strength. She, too, was with me but it was still terrifying.

A team came in, yanked out the Hickman, and left. It was incredibly painful. But sure enough, that turned out to be the source of the infection. My fever went away. Though it had been placed in my chest to deliver the chemo, the Hickman made the morning and evening blood draws quick and painless. Now that it was gone, they had to poke me with a needle for *every single blood draw*. At least twice a day.

148

It was traumatizing. Anxiety-filled moments each and every time. Another down side of chemo is that it makes your veins shrink, so they're harder to find. My nurses were rock stars at helping patients fight leukemia, but drawing blood wasn't something they did very often.

The first person to attempt a blood draw missed my vein, again and again. It was so stressful. I was so traumatized. The only one in the unit I trusted was a nurse named Kristy, who was already a specialist in needle placement of PICC lines which go in a patient's arms (in addition to treating leukemia). Don't you know I got out of bed every day looking for her? I checked the schedule and, if she wasn't there, asked when she would be back. I tried to laugh it off with the other nurses, but it made me so anxious!

They'd never be able to put the Hickman back, because of the infection risk. Instead, they finally inserted a PICC line—a catheter running from a vein in my upper arm to another in my chest—so I wouldn't have to be stuck.

Waiting for ZERO

Through it all, I walked and cried and puked and never let up. My counts dropped and hit rock bottom—that was the goal. I was a neutropenic. Next, I would count the days while my white cells climbed back up, this time slower than the last round. My numbers would climb, then drop, then climb. I was getting closer to Gabriel, but I was beaten down and running out of steam. It took almost three fearful, tearful weeks for my counts to climb back to a safe level.

At last, it was time to get on the phone to book flights for Cesar to go to Atlanta, get my mom and Gabriel, and bring them home. Southwest Airlines was amazing. Because we never knew when I'd be ready, I couldn't make cheaper reservations in advance: we were looking at sky-high last-minute fares. But I would call Southwest to explain, and beg for a decent rate, and each time I was met with awesome kindness. A representative would put me through to a manager, then help me work out the ticketing—never once charging us the higher price for same-day booking. No other airline would make special arrangements for us, not even Delta Airlines where my dad had worked for more than thirty years as a flight dispatcher. I'll always be indebted to Southwest for being so helpful in the worst of times.

Break #2

Gabriel was going to come! *Would he remember me?*

Barely. It was another heartbreaking moment of confusion. It took him a few days to warm back up to me. My poor son was so confused. And he hated having me wear a mask around him to protect against germs. But Alison, my psychologist-advisor in Austin, made a brilliant suggestion: Get him his own mask! I did, and he loved that.

In the two weeks or so that I was home, we made the most of our time, taking into account my risk of infection. We took Gabriel to petting zoos, pony rides, and face painting. Lots of hand sanitizer was involved. I knew I was playing with fire, but I so wanted to *live* and feel normal again, just for a little bit of time. By day we made memories, and at night my child fell asleep in

150

my arms, or on my chest. I wanted time to stand still. This poor little boy had no idea it would all soon end and I would be leaving him *again*.

His birthday had passed but we celebrated it a few days late. The date didn't matter. It mattered that I was there, ALIVE, and celebrating my son turning two. I'll never forget his smile and the picture we took on the steps of our home. He was my boy. I was his mom. Forever.

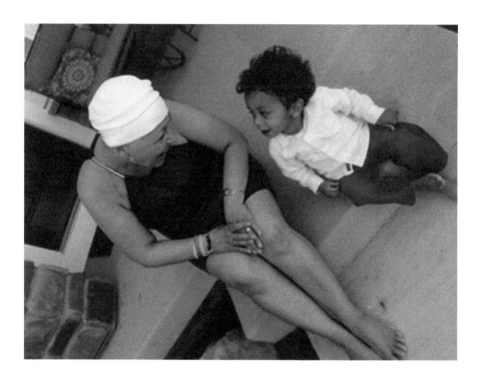

Somehow, God aligned this short break to allow me to celebrate two memory-making days at the same time—his birthday and Mother's Day. What an honor and privilege to be home and be alive to celebrate that day with my son and Cesar and my own mom. This wasn't just any day. This was MY day. And while moms usually say they aren't doing a damn thing on that day, they want to leave the house and go away, I wanted to do all things mom. I wanted to be the mom I couldn't be while in the hospital. I wanted the chaos in the house. I wanted to make breakfast. I wanted to do the dishes. I wanted to play with my son. I wanted to be exhausted with life of being a mom and celebrate my few days of freedom. Oh, how sweet it was!

This time when the break was over, I couldn't say goodbye. I tried. Gabriel was screaming, "Mommy, noooo. . . nooooo! Don't go, Mommy. Don't go!" But I knew I had to. What choice did I have? If I gave in, I would see him temporarily and then die from the disease. I had no other option. I had to suck it up. I had to put faith over fear. I had to believe in something bigger. I had to believe I was going to be the exception and get out of there alive. . . even if that meant another goodbye.

So, I did the absolute worst thing: After I got my son busy on a painting project, I walked out of the house without a word. Just fucking walked out of the house! Walked out. Yep. No farewell kiss, nothing. I was SO angry. I didn't know how to say goodbye. I couldn't handle the pain and looking in his eyes and lying again and saying, "Mommy is going to the store. I'll be right back." The lies, the pain, the trauma—they haunted me. What if that was the last time I ever was with him?

Cycle 3 - Cesar DROP- OFF this Time

Cesar drove me back to Johns Hopkins for my third cycle of chemo, ready to fight again. It was a long quiet drive. I wanted to punch a wall. I was speechless. It was like a scene out of a movie as I watched the world pass by as we drove. I was numb. My body was shaken to the core. I had just walked out on my son without saying goodbye. The guilt. My heart sank. How could I do that to him just because I didn't feel strong enough to cope with another tearful goodbye? To this day, he says he remembers wandering the house and looking for me and kept saying I had just disappeared on him. He didn't let me out of his sight for months, and to this day, he worries when I leave.

Back to the car ride to Hopkins. It was May. Once again, I rolled up with my giant suitcase, packed with everything I needed to ArmorUp against leukemia; workout gear and weights, but this time my Vitamix blender as well. I didn't care if it wasn't allowed in the hospital. I was going to fuel my body for success, making my own meal replacement drinks—with organic ingredients, not processed. Take that, cancer! Plus, I wasn't about to drink the processed shakes they had in the hospital fridge. You couldn't even pronounce the ingredients in those drinks. I long for the day we can give cancer patients the clean eating meals they truly need to "meet the medicine halfway."

Cesar checked me in and made sure I got settled in. Then he turned around and drove back to Virginia. There, he picked up Gabriel and my mom to escort them on the flight back to Atlanta, where this time he'd stay the whole weekend. Cesar booked an early flight home from Atlanta and he too never forgets how he didn't get to say goodbye. Cesar never forgave himself for that decision. It haunts him to this day. We handled this so poorly, but then again, who was advising us? There was no therapist from the hospital to help. No one. Psycho-oncology needs to be more than just an emerging field. It can't just be a term we throw around to make ourselves feel good like we are making progress. We need to actually have programs in place to help patients handle problems like this on the emotional level.

After my initial cycle of treatment, when Mom and Gabriel visited us the first time, Cesar accompanied them to Atlanta, then rushed back to Hopkins to be with me. By now, we had come to realize that Gabriel had been suffering in a way his little mind couldn't understand, and he needed more of his dad too—not just me. I would have to rise above my own needs and be strong alone, for now. This time it was Cesar's turn, when Sunday afternoon came, to make the tough getaway, saying goodbye with tears in his eyes. I know it broke his heart.

In fact, by this point Cesar and I had decided he would fly down to spend every other weekend with Gabriel. We were broke. Our charge cards were maxed, but we just charged on other cards. There was no amount of money that was going to come between Cesar and Gabriel. We would do anything to minimize his suffering. My mom would call crying, begging him to find the money to buy more tickets to see Gabriel. Our son was clearly struggling and needed him. It meant the husband I leaned on was away even more, and the little time I had to be with him was instead going to be with Gabriel, but I had to rise above that.

I would be alone even more for my fight, but that was the best we could do. I knew he was going to be with our son, but yet I would sit crying and screaming like a lunatic saying, *what about me? I need you. I sit alone in here staring at these four walls all day while you work. I'm alone. I have no daily caregiver. I need you.* But at that moment, I knew I had to once again put my head before my heart and focus on Gabriel and his well-being, and my husband who needed to see his son too. What a nightmare this was becoming.

Compounding Physical Effects

Back at the Sydney Kimmel Cancer Center, it was time to put another *damn calendar* on the wall and start this shit all over again: seven to ten days of toxic chemotherapy, then watch my blood counts fall and feel myself deteriorate, then fight to hold it together while my counts built back up to something approaching normal.

Each and every chemo dose compounded the one before it. Although this was a new treatment cycle, with a new calendar on the wall, nothing about it was new to my poor body. It was taking a beating, along with my heart. The time it took for me to respond physically to the drugs got longer and longer as treatment progressed. That's how it goes—and it can take months. Everything depends on how your body breaks down and builds back up.

Which, of course, depends on how you *prepare* and *present!*

Walk & Walk . . . Regrets

At that point, it felt like all I could do to help my outcome was walk and walk and walk. If I was going to die, at least it wouldn't be from pneumonia! Occasionally, I would beg the nurses to clean the tubing of my IV, which would set me free to walk without the IV stand. On one of those days I actually walked a total of 7.8 miles when I added it all up. Some days I wanted to keep going, out the doors of Johns Hopkins, and never look back.

As I shuffled along, the sicker I got, and the more my mind flashed on memories of my life and how I'd lived it. You know what went through my head? *Regrets. Every single one of them.*

I longed to have my freedom back—so I could do the things I didn't do when I was free to do them. I wanted to revisit each time my actions said *no* to things I wish I'd said *yes* to. I wanted to:

- Spend more time laughing and less time stressing out about things that, in the end, didn't matter.
- Find balance in my career, enjoying the now.
- Focus more on *real* problems, not first-world problems.
- Be with friends and loved ones instead of working overtime, all the time.
- Go on vacation, instead of banking days of vacation.
- Make more memories with my husband and son.
- Visit family more often.

Cesar/Care-taking

My husband slept at my side at the hospital that entire year, driving nearly an hour and a half each way to an extended workday in between, except on Sunday nights. A few months into my treatment, we agreed that he should go home to Northern Virginia each week (when he wasn't in Georgia with

Gabriel) and get a break from being on 24/7. Sit and relax. Watch football, run a load of laundry, take a shower in a *real* shower. Outline his week ahead so he could be focused and at the top of his professional game.

My husband is an introvert and also very private. He doesn't like asking for help. He internalizes everything and keeps things to himself. In fact, he didn't even tell our new neighbors what was going on. They would introduce themselves; he would say hi, and then go inside to get more clothes for the week. They had no idea I was fighting for my life thousands of miles away from my support system. His poker face never let on that he was dying inside with heartache.

Cesar worked full-time and then some. He put in his usual "half days" (which means 12 hours in the TV world!). He needed work. He needed to maintain his career. He needed it as an escape. We needed it to pay our bills and for insurance. We made it work. What choice did we have?

Many times, when Cesar was "off-duty" as a caregiver, my friend Tracey Garcia would come to spend the night. At the time she was a FOX News Network makeup artist and would come on her off days to spend the day with me, sleep next to me, clean up my throw up, hold my hand, listen to me cry, and yes, even make me feel pretty by doing my make up like I was about to go live! I'll never forget her kindness.

I'd made my career in broadcasting. I knew that my husband couldn't afford to carry his family's crisis into a high-pressure network management job. The news never stops, remember? His was our only salary now, and we had no other health insurance. We didn't want a single colleague at his office to complain he wasn't focused. In fact, he was *hyper*-focused. Cesar would call me briefly each day just to check in, and I had no doubt he would be there in an instant if I asked him to come. But I couldn't do that. He needed his career. We needed his benefits. We needed to pay our bills. Cesar's career, money, and health insurance were the driving force.

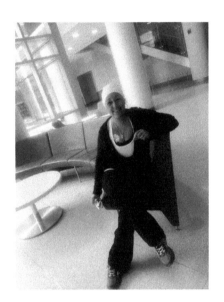
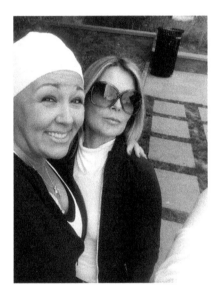

It was partly on me to help ensure that Cesar's career thrived, even in the face of our adversity. I encouraged him to attend events that might involve networking. Even on Easter Sunday! A girl who had started a meal train for us—to keep Cesar fed, along with all of us when I was home between treatment cycles—called me to invite him along to church, explaining that her terrific congregation was also a good place to make connections. Oh, okay, fine. I sent him off.

It sounded good in theory—until I found myself all alone and in tears on Easter, with no one to visit me. Out my window I saw smiling families walking into the hospital with flowers, or sitting outside with their loved ones. There I was in bed with MRSA, a drug-resistant staph infection, sitting on my ASS! I was in so much pain that I couldn't even walk down to the chapel to pray. I couldn't sit. I was so sad and disappointed in myself. Why had I suggested that my husband go? I wanted to support his career any way I could, but it turned out I had my limits.

When dear Tracey heard I was alone, she got in her car and drove all the way from Northern Virginia to be with me. She brought me flowers and then did my makeup again and took pictures. Yes, despite my pain and everything else swirling around me, she made me feel beautiful for an hour—long enough to forget about my troubles.

Most times, there was no one to fill the void. I spent *thousands* of in-patient hours without someone to sit with me and hold my hand, the way others on the floor seemed to have constant company. I so longed for human touch, but between the germs and my risk of bruising and bleeding, I couldn't be held or hugged, kissed or caressed. Even the medical massage therapist we eventually hired (I charged that too!!) had to wear protective gloves, and since my platelet count made me prone to bruising, her touch was minimal.

I cried a lot. I was angry at the world.

It might hurt Cesar to read this, but the point is that in many ways I fought my battle by myself, while he fought another one. I know I was never alone, because he walked the journey with me, every day. But he had a job we all depended on. Professionally and financially, it seemed to be our family's only way through. I put aside my desperate need for companionship...and yet my strategy of suffering in silence didn't really work.

Other Patients—Concealment

I realize that, with my daily posts to my **ArmorUp** for LIFE® community on social media, it doesn't sound like I was all that silent. It seems like I put it all out there, but in practice I only mostly shared. *I withheld some of my pain and suffering* to protect my husband and his career. I had to.

It's true, I was able to connect with thousands of people in the outside world by reporting on my experience through social media and TV segments I researched. This inspired others to join my fight and ArmorUp.

For some leukemia patients in our ward, though, that kind of openness was unimaginable. I had friends on the floor who clearly were suffering, yet they'd post online about how great they felt and how well their days was going. I was shocked. Others never told a soul they had cancer. They kept it secret, to safeguard their jobs, their ability to earn an income, and their opportunity to provide for their families. You can't blame them.

It breaks my heart that these fellow patients felt the need to hide reality from their own friends and loved ones. And if the world at large can't fully grasp the impact of this hell we call cancer, how can we build support for better care and research? Our fight and our stories need to be out there. They need to resonate and make an impact so we can change the course of treatment for those who follow in our footsteps.

SURVIVOR Moment

I remember taking a walk through the hospital one weekend when Cesar was with me. In the lobby we happened to pass an event for survivors. Turns out, they considered me to be one. Who knew?

I was beaten down, holding onto my husband's arm, struggling to put one foot in front of the other. When the lady at the table handed me a 6-Month Survivor Button, I cried and said, "I'm not a survivor yet! I'm still fighting, and I feel like the finish line is getting pushed further and further away."

After ongoing breathing difficulties, weakness, pain and exhaustion, my counts were finally on the rebound—slower than the last round, but moving in the right direction. Soon it was time for me to scramble and book airline tickets so Cesar could bring my mom and Gabriel back for a visit.

The good news, I found out you are a survivor from the day of your diagnosis.

Break #3: Surgery and Self-Driving

Cesar drove both Gabriel and my mom straight to Hopkins and waited near the lobby elevator to greet me. This time it was a quiet reunion. Gabriel, now two years old, was still confused, but he held me tight and didn't want to let go. It filled my heart, even while the unknown future tormented me. So many of my friends with cancer had died and left their children. They loved them just as much as I loved Gabriel. I wanted a guarantee it wouldn't happen to me, but that's not how life works. The only thing to do was enjoy the moment, so when we got home, I laid down on the couch and held my little boy tight.

As if things weren't complicated enough, Gabriel needed surgery to remove his tonsils and adenoids. My mom had reported that, at night, when her grandson slept next to her, she'd worry that his breathing levels were poor. During my previous break at home the doctor who evaluated his condition had urged us to address it as soon as possible.

The very next day, we were off to a different hospital, for Gabriel. I thought my heart would explode. It was just too much. The surgery nurses insisted I should go home because there were too many germs floating around, but *no way* was I leaving my boy. They saw me walk in with my N95 mask and got worried. They insisted a germy hospital—a pediatric unit especially—was no place for an immune-compromised patient. But I wasn't going anywhere. Nope! How could I NOT be there for my son after I had abandoned him for so long?

Gabriel had his operation and spent the night at the hospital. And at six o'clock the very next morning I got in the car and headed back to Hopkins for testing and treatment follow-ups. It was just for the day, but it exhausted me. Cesar had to stay home to take care of Gabriel, so *I drove myself.*

I look back and think how crazy and dangerous that was, me barreling along the highway with low platelets and little sleep. Not to mention that I had no one else along to confirm what the medical staff told me, and to understand how critical the information was and what the next steps should be. Crazier still, I've driven myself to scores of check-ups since then. There has got to be a better way.

Cycle 4

Yes, there was a Cycle 4. It seemed to go on and on. Let's just say it was even harder, and even longer . . . It was taking a toll on me and everyone around me trying to hold it together. We were going broke and I was feeling broken. Another 7+3-day chemo regimen. Another round of killing cells and letting them rebuild and another round of the waiting game, hoping and praying.

When my counts were at a safe level, Dr. Levis set me free. He said, "This is all we can do for you. Go make memories. Live your best life. Celebrate each moment. We can't do anything else for you."

I wasn't sure what that meant. But I packed up my big suitcase from those four sterile white walls of 5B leukemia unit room and headed home and into Gabriel's arms with my N95 mask and my heart full.

In my mind I was healed!

Three days later, I got the call.

I heard the words, "You have cancer" yet a second time.

CHAPTER 10

Transplant

I will never forget the phone call I got one October day while trying to make memories with my son. I wanted to look into his eyes and say I was home for good and that Mommy would never leave him again, but something made me scared to say it. I was scared it wasn't the truth. I couldn't even get the nerve up to unpack my suitcase once and for all. I had hurriedly packed it one too many times this year for emergencies and then my fifty-day hospital stays.

I should have unpacked by then. I was home from the hospital after ten months of fighting leukemia. They had sent me home and said that was it. There was nothing else they could do for me. They thought the remission would hold, but there was no guarantee. I had done those four rounds of HDAC (ten months) and I was told my body had maxed out on the amount of chemo I could physically handle. At some point, the chemo can kill you instead of the cancer. It is simply THAT toxic. There was and still is no official cure for leukemia, so I was rightly hesitant and scared.

I wasn't supposed to be out in public because of my mask and risk of germs, but I wanted to get out of the house and start making memories so we did. We were having a blast, laughing, giggling, running after each other when I looked down at my phone and saw that my oncologist was calling me. FROM HIS CELL PHONE at 4:00 PM in the afternoon. My heart sank. Holy shit! What happened? Why is he calling me?

I answered the phone with my lip trembling and my heart racing ninety miles an hour. "Hello. Dr. Levis?"

He said, "Hi Loriana, I need to meet with you and your husband tomorrow morning at 8:00 AM. I need both of you there. We need to have a talk."

"OMG, OMG . . . please Dr. Levis, talk to me. What is it? Tell me it's not back? Pleasssssssseee."

I began to scream into the phone and drown out every child screaming in the entire place. It was like the first time I heard those words. "You have cancer." It all came back to me and the room started to spin.

I grabbed Gabriel and ran out the door. I put him in the car and I told Dr. Levis to give me more information and all he would say was, "Your cancer is coming back and we will need to move fast. Decisions need to be made quickly. I will see you at 8:00 AM."

Holy shit! No, dear GOD, why? Why the fuck is this happening to me? Can I get a break? My son needs me. I'm so tired. I want off this fucking ride.

So, I call my husband screaming like a lunatic. Gabriel is now screaming and crying too. I tell him I need him home now and scream in the most terrifying high-pitched sound you can imagine. Cesar gets home an hour later to find me sobbing on the couch, holding Gabriel and hysterical. He holds me and we pray. Then we dry our tears and start making action plans. Start building our pit crew, yet again. Nothing had been discussed, but we knew the steps. Transplant was next. If that didn't work, death was a possibility option. How the hell was this happening?

The next morning at 6:00 AM we carried Gabriel into our neighbors' home while I cried. He barely knew this family, but what choice did I have? I kissed him a million times. I was scared they were going to check me in that day and not let me out. I packed my bags, just in case. All the fears and worries again. "What if I die and don't see him again? What if I don't find a match? Where am I going to find 100 caregivers for 100 days? How will my husband keep his job?"

We got to Johns Hopkins and rushed into Dr. Levis's office and this is how he explained it. He said, "You need a transplant and you need one soon. The bone marrow clinical trial you were a part of found your cancer coming back. We suspected something was happening because it has been almost eighty days now since we knocked your counts down with chemo and you still haven't built yourself back up. AND . . . thankfully this test confirmed it before it was too late. This test looks at the baby cells before they grow up to full-blown cancer. But we also need to move quickly. You technically are STILL in remission, but you won't be for long and once you come out of remission it will be too hard to fight."

I cried and asked, "What can happen if I come out of remission before a transplant?"

Dr. Levis explained, "You will likely succumb to the disease and die."

"What? How?" I fired back these two questions in rapid succession.

He explained, "Well you MUST be in remission to have a transplant. If you come out of remission then I have to do induction again and go through another forty to fifty-day cycle and then go into transplant, but most people don't make the second induction. It is too hard on the body and you already took too long to recover from the last round, so it wouldn't look good."

My husband held my hand and we both, without a doubt, said we would absolutely move forward despite the risk of death. I mean, what fucking choice did we have? Either way I chose, risk of death was an option.

Thank GOD I had taken part in that LLS (Leukemia & Lymphoma Society) funded study. Holy shit! It was about to potentially save my life. The way this study worked was by looking deeper into the bone marrow, at the baby cells. Today, when you have a painful bone marrow biopsy, they pull marrow out and doctors are able to assess the mature cells and say, "yes you have a blood cancer," or "no you don't," and then go from there. This study is so remarkable because it is able to look at the baby cells BEFORE they grow up and mature so doctors can take swift action and treat patients before they come out of remission and before the cancer comes back. Amen. But this study wanted to randomize me and my doctor and I weren't going to allow that. I had a two-and-a-half-year-old waiting for me. Dr. Levis pulled me out of the study. We got the answer we needed and then started down the road of preparing for transplant. We had so many more questions and Dr. Levis was patient and answered, and he never minced words. He was transparent even if it was painful.

On another note, I wish all patients had access to this study. I wish I still had access to this study. Who wouldn't want to detect the cancer cells while they are babies before they develop back into full-blown blasts of cancer—before it's tougher to treat, or possibly too late? THIS is why we need more funding so this type of test can be fast-tracked and approved for EVERY ONE OF US . . . not just those in the study and those agreeing to be randomized. I knew it was an amazing test when I signed up for the study and I had full intentions of receiving my answer and getting out of the study.

Next step, finding my match. My sister was my perfect match, but she had a heart murmur and they weren't sure from a legal standpoint they would allow her to save my life, even if it meant me dying because of it. They couldn't kill my sister trying to save me. They simply could not risk putting two lives in danger. I asked him, "What happens if my sister can't save me then? What next?" I was always used to a Plan B. In TV, every reporter has a backup and a backup to their backup for the big story.

Dr. Levis said, "You will likely succumb to the disease and die. The bone marrow donor registry is 70 percent Caucasian and you are mixed race. This is very tough to find, and we are in a race against time."

It was so raw to hear that. Just plain RAW! I started shaking. I began praying for my sister to be healthy enough to save my life. I've never been so grateful for her matching love for fitness and bootcamps.

Then we met with the transplant coordinator, Katheryn Yarcony and I started learning the facts.

- My sister had to fly up here immediately and begin two weeks of medical testing and clearances. That included physical and psychological testing.
- Once I start my transplant, they would need me for 100 days.
- My insurance would ONLY cover the actual transplant process. That meant the process of retrieving my sister's bone marrow and me receiving it, and the treatment surrounding it, but not my hospital stays. I would have to pay out of pocket to sleep in their attached housing for other transplant patients in the same situation. The cost was $120 a night, plus parking, food, etc. for the caregiver.
- Nothing was covered except my daily visits to see the doctors but no hospital stays and Johns Hopkins prides itself on success rates and if you want a transplant with them, you MUST be on site, live nearby or prove you are staying at a local hotel. I support them on this decision. This is why Johns Hopkins is known for its high standards. They want to make sure that if you get a fever that you can get help in thirty minutes, because when you are neutropenic and have no immune system that can mean life or death. I'm so glad we stayed there on site, but it did cost $10,000 in housing alone, plus the housing supplies, food, etc. Each day we went deeper into debt.
- I needed a caregiver for EVERY SINGLE DAY, 24/7, or I would get kicked out. Where the hell was I going to find 100 people?

There's almost what appears to be something like a separation of church and state with the transplant. You have your team of doctors and then a transplant team that handles the process. Your doctor is not allowed to influence or approve your sister for transplant. The transplant team has to decide IF it is safe for her, not if it is good for me.

The transplant team set up my sister's tests, and she flew up here. We started the testing. I remember sitting outside the room for each of her tests. One of those tests included a meeting with the legal department to ask again and get legal clearance that she did in fact want to go through with this. It would be painful. She could lose a lot of blood. She could die trying to save me. It was going to be hard on her and they needed to assess her mental state to feel confident she would not walk away in mid-transplant before the actual transfer. It had happened before. Doctors had done all the prep chemo days, killed off all the cells for a patient, got them ready to accept the marrow, and their loved one or donor got scared and left, ultimately leaving the cancer patient high and dry.

I begged my sister, "Just go in and agree to everything. Say yes to whatever. Please, please, help me." I could tell she was scared. But my son needed his mother. I knew she had ArmoredUp (for LIFE) her entire life. She was fit for this fight.

Then we went to take the EKG. Again, I wasn't allowed in the testing room. I heard the beeping. I heard them say it was not a regular heartbeat. The person administering the EKG came out and I said, "Please do it again. She's okay, right? Look, she's fit. She does boot camps.

They in turn said to me, "We just do the test. Take this to your doctor."

I cried the entire way over to see the doctor. I kept asking myself, *what does this murmur, low heart rate mean to me? What does it mean to my life?* We delivered the test to the doctor in the other building who managed and approved transplants, and then we waited and waited. Needless to say, I cried the entire time. One test after another over this two-week period had stressed me out. And all this time I'm also thinking, "Hurry up! *If I come out of remission I'm totally screwed. Why does this have to take so long?"* All along I knew the transplant team had so many safety and legal measures it needed to take, but at the time none of that rational information mattered to me. This was also precious time with Gabriel that I was missing out on.

While my sister met with the transplant team, I was speaking with the transplant coordinator about the other matches they might have found on the national database. There was no match for me. No one of Cuban/Italian descent with my genetic makeup had signed up. The way it was explained is that my human leukocyte antigen, or HLA, must match someone on the registry. HLA is your protein or marker, found on most cells in your body. HLA types are inherited, and you are more likely to match someone with your ancestry which is why they test your family first but look for back-ups on the registry. Many people depend on the registry and complete strangers to save their lives. So, I asked what happened if my sister wasn't cleared, and their faces told the story. In a nutshell, if there was no match, then I would likely succumb to the disease and die.

What? WTF? You mean that's it? This was all so stressful. My friends were holding swab parties and drives in an all-out effort to find my match. But it was explained to me that even if they did succeed in their endeavor, the process would take so long that it wouldn't help me now but it could save others in the future. *Good,* I thought. *Let's boost the registry and the number of its minority donors. It is desperately needed.*

Back to my sister. The doctor came out and called her name so that the final decision could be made. She needed to be told the risks involved and her medical tests had to be assessed. He also needed to measure how confident she sounded about saving my life. Was she really committed and willing to see this through? I literally followed the doctor to the point of stalking him. He turned around and told me that I wasn't allowed to go in. "This is a private conversation."

With tears in my eyes, I said, "Please pass her. My son needs me. Please, I don't have another match." I can't imagine how often the transplant team hears these kinds of pleas. It is truly heartbreaking.

An hour later, my sister walked out, hugged me, smiled, and said, "We're in. I'm going to save your life." I'm crying as I am writing these words. OMG! Even now I feel so honored. All I could do when my sister gave me the good news was cry because I felt so blessed. I had met several people who were waiting for a match so there was no way I was taking my sister's special gift to me for granted.

Next, they had to schedule my transplant, so they sent me home to prepare and get bags packed. I also had to find 100 days of caregivers and say goodbye to Gabriel, yet again. This was going to be the longest stretch without him. After having sat through the required informational transplant class, I also knew that it could very well be the last time I saw him if things didn't go well.

So, there I was at my kitchen table. All I wanted to do was hold my son and play with him, but instead I found myself in a panic creating a spreadsheet, running "Operation Transplant" and calling everyone I knew to be a caregiver. I was going to need 100 days of caregiving. I had just moved to the area and only knew about five people, and them not even all that well. I kept asking myself: Who can take time off work and fly here to stay with me? Can family members each take a week to help me out? Who can just pick up and leave their family and friends to care for someone for an entire week?

In order to begin the transplant process, I had to assure my team that I had all 100 days of caregiving covered. With all this drama going on, I made calls like I was running a political phone bank, freaking out and praying that I didn't come out of remission because then it would be over. Adding more to my anxiety was the countless studies that showed the impact of stress on the body can also cause cancer progression.

I had no choice but to go into reporter mode with tunnel vision. With one mission in mind, I placed call after call. "How are you? I'm okay. Listen, I need a transplant. Do you think you can take a week off work and come take care of me 24/7?" The entire time I was sobbing and only one could really understand me.

I also tried the following, "Hi, how are you? I have a calendar on Google Docs. You said you could help out. Which date can you take?" I was booking people for six, eight, and twenty-four hour shifts, and weeks at a time. It was complete nuts.

My mom was taking care of my son in Georgia so I couldn't ask her to be a caregiver. My sister was going to be busy saving my life so she couldn't be one either. As for my dad, he wasn't that well physically. Technically, he could have been a caregiver, even if I ended up having to take care of him. That actually happened; I pushed him around in the wheelchair. But at least there was someone with a pulse in the room so they didn't cancel my transplant. If something happened to him, we would be close to a hospital.

I called cousins and friends, and as much as they wanted to help, most of them couldn't just pick up and leave their jobs. To make matters worse we had ZERO money to pay for a full-time caregiver. I didn't really need a nurse. I needed *anyone* with a pulse. Someone breathing who could push me in a wheelchair to the main hospital when I went downhill in an instant. Someone to call my nurse and say I had a fever and would need help now. Of course, someone who knew and cared about me would be nice too, but at that point all I needed was a human being . . . *any* human being.

Thankfully, after hustling on the phone for days, I found earth angels to take care of me. The only sad part was that I had to go into reporter mode and did not have a single moment to hold my son, which is what I had cried about for months to be able to do. Fortunately, I was able to piecemeal 100 days of caregivers! Yes, 100 days! I was the miracle worker.

In fact, later that day I was in the driveway talking to some dear neighbors who had a friend coming to town—a Cuban woman named JoAnn. We had an instant connection. She got out of the car smiling and happy to be visiting with her friends. I immediately shared my story in the driveway, tears rolling down my face. As I cried, I joked and said, "Want to take a day?"

"Oh my God!" she exclaimed. "Sign me up for three weeks!"

Talk about there being angels among us. Sometimes you just have to wave the white flag and ask for help. Later I learned that she, too, had gone through a time in life that she needed others to care for her. She had always wanted the opportunity to pay that moment forward. She sure did!

I was able to finish filling out my spreadsheet with a few friends who took one or two days here and there. A cousin of mine signed up for a week, JoAnn for another. My father filled in the holes for two weeks. Cesar took a vacation week for Thanksgiving and Christmas. That's how we were able to make it happen.

The next day, I had to leave Gabriel. Going back to the hospital with Cesar for a transplant class was the last thing I wanted to do. They put me in a room with about ten other patients, and a nurse walked us through the entire transplant process. The only problem was, she opened up the class with each of us introducing ourselves and saying why we were there, what kind of transplant we were getting, who our match was. We didn't even make it all the way around the room before three patients spoke up and said, "Hi I'm _____ and I'm here for my second transplant because my first one didn't work. They had to find me another match."

WHAT? I got up and left the class. I was done. I thought the transplant was going to be the answer to my prayers. Why the HELL would they put new transplant patients looking for hope and the closest thing to a cure in a room with those who had undergone the procedure only to have it fail miserably? What a way to walk into a transplant. If your mind plays such an important role in your success . . . this was a shitty way to start us off. AND . . . I knew I had no backup. This made zero sense to me. Cesar stayed for the entire class. Everyone else looked unmoved. Either they were able to control their emotions well or they were in much better mental states than I was. I couldn't handle it. This messed with my head. I kept asking myself, "What if I fail? What is next?" Up until then, I had it in my head that it was all going to work out.

BEING THE VOICE

Proud moment I later spoke at Johns Hopkins through ArmorUp for LIFE's advocacy work and that transplant class is now split up between those going through their first transplant and those going through their second.

After the class, we went back home. My husband got back to his job and I spent time just holding my son and making a list of what I needed to pack for my apartment-style living. I was on a waiting list to stay in Johns Hopkins out-patient housing, a place called Hackerman which is similar to a Ronald McDonald house only it costs $120 a night. Sure, it was cheaper than a hotel and connected to the hospital, but with 100 nights the bill was still going to be a whopping $12,000.

I had to bring my own supplies: sheets, bedding, cooking utensils, outlet adapters, a mop to clean the floors (housekeeping had to be done once a week and you are at a high risk of infection), cleaning supplies, laundry detergent, shower mats, bathroom rugs, toothpaste, paper plates, and a big dry-erase board to keep up with my forty-plus medications and times so that my caregiver could help me remember what to take and when. There was not going to be a nurse held responsible for my daily medicine intake. Daily visits to the hospital were for follow-ups and other treatments only and not my pill intake.

My sister and I headed out to start gathering supplies, but nothing mattered more than finding a Christmas tree. As my doctor suggested, we were going to put the tree up now and take pictures with Gabriel so I could make the memories with him to save and have . . . *just in case*. Just in case I didn't make it. It is almost hard to process those words and even type them. How crazy it is, but it's true. If I died, Gabriel needed these pictures of me. Isn't that awful? I swore that if I survived, we would put up our Christmas tree every year on October 16th. It is now part of our family tradition. Oddly enough, that is also our anniversary date.

I held Gabriel in my arms and we decorated the tree. Every head turn, every reach to hang an ornament, every giggle, every movement, I snapped a picture with tears rolling down my face. Gabriel would look at me and take his little hands to my eyes and keep drying them and kissing me. He had no idea what was about to happen but he knew something wasn't right.

After that, we got in the car and headed to a family farm in northern Virginia to make some memories. Looking back, I can honestly say I was crazy. There I was, immune-compromised, an N-95 mask on, a port in my chest with a catheter tube attached, going down slides with my son on a burlap blanket. I was exhausted mentally and physically, but we were about to make more memories and act like life was perfect. Soon it was time for me to go. We booked Cesar and Gabriel's ticket on Southwest (the BEST & only airline who helped us with discounted rates) so he could take our son back to Atlanta to my mom. The time came to say goodbye. Except for loss itself, it was the worst pain a mother could feel—saying goodbye and not knowing if I would ever see him again.

I cried and did exactly the same thing I had done during my previous goodbyes; I lied. "Mommy is going to the store. You are going back to see Nana," I said to Gabriel.

He screamed and yelled. "Mommy! Mommy! I want Mommy!" Cesar had to pry him off of me so they wouldn't miss their flight. To this day when he cries and says, "Mommy! Mommy! Mommy!" I have horrible flashbacks.

Cesar would fly Gabriel to Atlanta with my sister, spend the day getting him settled, and then come back to get me for the drive to Hopkins to check me in at the Hackerman Outpatient Facility. Then, for the next 100 days, my full-time job was to survive. I would be at the hospital from 8:00 AM until 7:00 PM and then at night retreat to my little apartment-style room with my caregiver. This is something no one really has any idea about. People seem to think having a transplant is like an overnight surgery—you check in, transfer the marrow, check out and *voila.* It's like magic and you feel like a superstar. This couldn't be further from the truth. It's the same story like the other rounds, only *more* and *different* petty torments to deal with. There is no way around the pop-up problems, but the goal is to skate through those 100 days with as few issues as possible so doctors can monitor if and how the bone marrow from your donor is settling.

I had to do a week to ten days of prep work for the transplant. That meant some very intense chemo and full-body radiation to completely wipe out my cells before my sister would be needed. Yes, full-body radiation. Not the "targeted" radiation you might get for a different type of cancer. My cancer was everywhere.

This was an insane amount of chemo in a very short time coupled with radiation. Radiation was one thing I didn't have to do the entire year for my fight. For radiation, you have to go twice. Once for radiation planning, where radiologists get the measurements of where the radiation is going to be targeted and then once to actually do the radiation. Either time, you CANNOT MOVE. To make it manageable, I took a Xanax to calm down and lie still. You must stay perfectly still because they have exact targets to hit. The planning session lasted an hour because they have to position the angles accurately so the rest of your body receives minimal impact.

Once I returned for the actual radiation, they put some heavy thing on me, put me alone in the dark room on the table, and next thing I knew the lasers were going every which way. I'm so glad I gave in and listened to them when my doctor suggested a Xanax to relax. As I mentioned before, I rarely caved in to anything that would make me a foggy version of myself for fear I would lose motivation to ArmorUp and start a vicious cycle I couldn't escape. This time, I needed it. Further proof of that: I also had chemo that day.

By the third of my 100 days, I was starting to feel the chemo and the radiation. Remember, it really wasn't just a day of chemo. It was eleven months of chemo, plus one day. My body had been taking a beating from chemo for almost eleven months now. I had no idea what official day of chemo I was on but it was hell. It was a violent beatdown.

Some days when things didn't go so well it turned into twelve or fourteen hours. It was my JOB. Everything worked just like being an in-patient, only I had to walk over from the other building because my insurance only covered the treatment. Not the stay. Ridiculous, I know. We spent more than ten thousand dollars in living arrangements alone. Not to mention the travel for caregivers, the food, parking and so much more.

Each day at 8:00 AM, I would have to check in upstairs on the fifth floor where I had battled leukemia my first ten months. I would have to walk over from my building to the cancer center, get blood work done, then go sit in a large treatment room with beds and curtains. Each room had a number and each day I was assigned to a place where doctors, physicians assistants, and nurses would treat me just as if I was an in-patient. They were long exhausting days. It was like reporting to work without knowing when or what was going to blow up. I mention crisis management a lot when I talk about my husband's job and TV news, but this was another form of crisis management.

When I was stable enough to go back to my Hackerman "apartment," I was only allowed to return with the assistance of my caregiver. I had to prove I had one there with me 24/7 or they could not continue treatment. Two days after all the chemo and radiation, my sister arrived to prepare for her bone marrow donor surgery. She came and slept in my room and hugged me. There were no words for my gratitude. I looked at her and cried. The next day was going to be my NEW birthday. I couldn't believe it.

I was going to get a second chance at LIFE.

A second chance to live the life I should have been living.

A second chance to be the best mom I could be.

It was time.

It was transplant day.

During the transplant the goal is for your donor's marrow to settle in your body, flex its muscle, and then suppress your marrow. During that part there is a fight expected. That fight shows up in the form of what's called GVHD, or Graft vs Host Disease. It is a fight that doctors WANT your body to have, but only strong enough to indicate the other marrow is winning. Too much of a fight can be fatal, and not enough it can mean the transplant didn't work. This is why doctors really have to monitor you and you can't leave. Fevers pop up, infections arise, breathing problems surface, and you struggle to just catch your breath. Lying down was impossible; I would gasp for air. Every single day was another torment and yet each day I was expected to try my best to ride out the storm. I was terrified about what may happen next. I heard the next patient's story on the other side of the curtain and I would wonder, what hell would I face next?

At 5:00 AM the next morning, Cesar and I walked my sister to her surgery. They hooked her up to IVs, read her info about the risks again, and I sobbed as they wheeled her back to surgery. It was so surreal. I couldn't believe such a miracle was about to take place and my hero was going to be my sister.

In this surgery they had to put the donor under full anesthesia for the time it would take to extract the amount of marrow needed to save my life. They had to go into my sister's marrow with that lovely instrument mentioned earlier in the book that looks like a corkscrew. The extraction is similar to a biopsy, but instead of one or two times of going into her marrow they went into her marrow 140 times. She lost so much blood she had to be admitted to the hospital for days to get transfusions and recover.

Even then, the stress isn't over yet. There are so many milestones that have to be met to call this a success. The first step is: the procedure *has* to go well. They have to be able to extract enough marrow to replace mine that was destroyed with the chemo. Then my marrow would have to accept it, allow it to replace it, and then allow it to stay in charge forever. There are a lot of factors.

Cesar and I waited and watched the monitors. I prayed. I was so stressed out. The doctors came out and my heart raced. I was sweating and one of them said, "We got the marrow." It was like a movie where a big theft takes place and they said, "We got the goods!" "Now we need to wait and see if we got enough for your transplant," the doctor added.

OMG! OMG! Praise the LORD. God is great. I was still on edge.

The doctor continued to brief us, "But your sister lost a lot of blood in the procedure; she's waking up and is in a lot of pain. She is going to need some blood transfusions and will have to spend the night in the hospital, NOT the outpatient center."

I was so worried. I worried that she wasn't going to be okay. When I finally got to see her, I just cried. She was smiling but in pain. All she said to me was, "I love you. I would do anything for you. I want you to raise your son and be home with Cesar and Gabriel."

How do you ever say thank you to someone for saving your life?

I followed my sister to her room. They checked her in and started her blood transfusions to replace all the blood loss from surgery. Once the collected marrow was cleaned and processed for me, it was my turn to receive the transplant. I went back to my treatment room, waited for nurses to arrive and finally they walked in with my LIFE literally in their hands . . . a

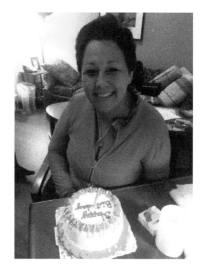

bag of marrow that looked just like a bag of blood. I thought it would look different. They wrapped a sling around it over and over again to make sure it didn't drop, they started the drip, and then my nurses did something so sweet—they sang "Happy Birthday." I had a cake and even took a picture to save for the rest of my life.

OCT 29, This Was My New Birthday

THIS was the day of my new life.

My life would forever change on this day. I would have to mourn who I once was and embrace who I would soon be . . . if I lived . . . to just be . . .

Doctors knew I worked well by setting goals and reaching milestones so they told me, "Your next goal: 100 days. The next 100 days will be hell, but how you get through them will be critical to your success or failure, and so many factors play a role."

So how did I manage the stress of trying to survive the first 100 days? It reminded me of how we tracked our President's progress during the first 100 days in office. These are the days the President has to make good on promises and really give it 150 percent and deliver. That was goal two. My promise was to inspire throughout my entire battle and realize this fight was bigger than me . . . it was about educating the public and being a transparent journalist and fitness/health reporter.

So, in the midst of all this craziness, what did I do? I challenged family, friends, viewers, and fans to do something again in my honor—to get fit on a number of different levels such as diet, exercise, meditation, financial fitness or spiritual. It was accountability on both sides. I made myself walk and stay positive and report back to them, and they reported to me on what they did to improve their lives and get prepared for whatever fight came their way.

Transplant Week

My dad took a turn staying with me. He wanted to be near both his daughters for the transplant and while we recovered. My sister stayed two nights in the hospital getting blood transfusions and getting stabilized while I stayed with my dad in the Hackerman Building. I wanted to sleep at my sister's side, but I also needed help and to be near my own nurses. Even in the midst of chaos, sisters will be sisters. My sister kept calling me to say she felt lonely in her room with no visitors and it was so scary. I looked at her like a deer caught in headlights and said, "What? Hello? Lonely? You spent a whole two days here with me coming in and out. Girl, let me check you in for a few months and then you'll see what loneliness and fear is really like."

After ten months as an in-patient with nurses running to my room for every *beep, beep, beep,* it was terrifying to know the high stakes of my transplant and to be in an apartment unit attached to the hospital with a caregiver who knew ZERO about cancer. I was terrified. I knew that I could die if I got a fever and didn't get immediate treatment. I knew the reality. There was a tunnel to walk through to get to the hospital, but cutting the cord of being on-site a bit was scary. I may have acted independent in the hospital, but the nurses were my security blanket. Now, I had to be my own security blanket. I still did my walks twice a day. I ate simply and cleanly each day. It was overwhelming to say the least.

Like I had done my entire life, I had to pull from my own strength once again. I was always the strong one in my family. I had to do it again, even under these most trying circumstances, to take care of myself. I ended up caring for my dad while he was staying as my caregiver. I ended up helping my sister as she recovered from the hospital. I have no idea how in the world I pulled this off, but again I had no choice. This is the situation my health insurance put me in. My dad doesn't cook, didn't know how to take care of me, but GOD bless him he tried. My sister was a mess emotionally and physically. It was at that moment, I realized how strong I had actually become over the course of ten months. I was used to hiding my pain and sucking it up. It's what I did. It is what I knew. I was also filled with gratitude (picture of me pushing my sister). I actually pushed my sister back and forth to the hospital in a wheelchair each day for her follow-up appointments and held my dad's hand, and *I* was the one who had the transplant. It took me back to my childhood, where I always felt I had to be stronger even in the times of weakness.

Once my sister and dad left, then it was a parade of caregivers of family members like my cousin Marylin, my step-mom Jane, my new rock-star friend Joann who I met in my neighbor's driveway, then my dad again, and we just kept rotating until Christmas. It was really tough having a caregiver sleep in my room and spend 24-7 with me each and every day. I couldn't run from my depression or hide it. Each day had small victories and defeats. I wanted to go on my walks alone and cry, but I couldn't go anywhere without someone at my side. I felt blessed to have them, but felt I had another layer of freedom taken away. And it was really overwhelming—forty-plus pills a day, each at different times, some with food, others two hours after food, some on an empty stomach. With so many different caregivers, I had to use my dry-erase board to stay on top of it.

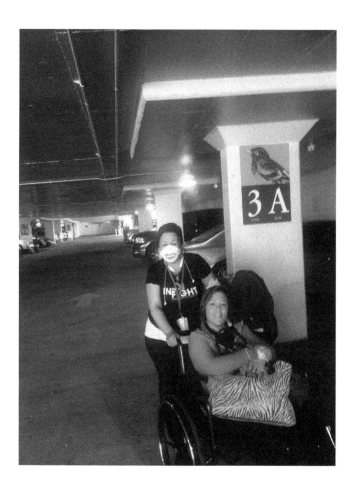

Then on the board I had to list what to take for headaches, what to take for nausea; for every scenario, I wrote down the response so in the event of an emergency, my caregiver knew what to do. I had unbelievable migraines, but they couldn't give me anything but caffeine pills because they couldn't mask a potential infection. I remember sitting up in bed at night crying and begging for help, but there was nothing they could do for me.

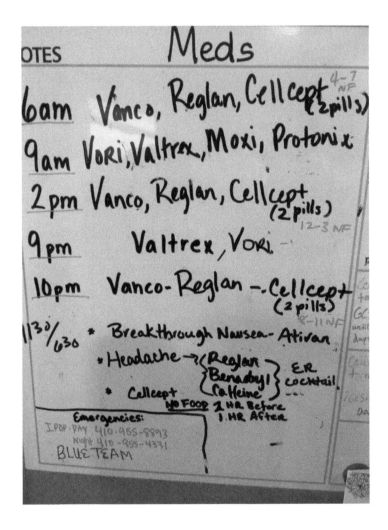

One of my caregivers, Jo Anne, is very much into meditation and would push me to meditate, and I would get angry. I would say, "I can't lie down and think and visualize. I can barely breathe when I lie down. I have a pounding headache."

I didn't want to do anything . . . I wanted cancer to go the fuck away. Then I would meditate, but at that very moment it wasn't going to work for me. As much as I love meditation, it was impossible to do any sort of breathing exercises because I could barely breathe. I couldn't sit still because if I did the pain felt worse and my mind would travel to death. It was best to just keep my mind busy or it would be the end of me.

Adding to my stress, every time I would FaceTime with Gabriel, he'd look at me, cry, and walk away. He didn't want to talk to me. It showed me how easily one could be forgotten. He was so young. He had just started to know life without me. It was an unbelievable pain in my heart all day long. It made me so angry at the world. To help me cope, my best friend Amy, the chief pit crew leader, would call and let me cry and then say, "Let's get to work; we have to get your website up and running." She would give me assignments each day to help her build the site. Like, "today you need to write the content about this tab." Then later in the day she would call me and we would work on creating my ArmorUp for LIFE® logo. Just like my news director Pam, Amy was doing what she could do to give me HOPE, and it worked.

Day 17

I lost my hair *again*! They promised me it would happen again. OMG, it just started growing back and I felt like I looked more feminine again and now it was falling out in big clumps.

GVHD (Graft vs Host Disease) was in full swing. The official definition, a condition that might occur *after* an allogeneic *transplant*. In GVHD, the donated *bone marrow* or peripheral blood stem cells view the recipient's body as foreign, and the donated cells *bone marrow* attack the body. As miserable as it was, that's a disease, according to Dr. Levis, you *want* to get. It's a sign of the bone marrows fighting. I was the host and my sister was the graft. The goal was to let it roar for some time to help boost my chances of survival, but the GVHD was an unbelievable type of misery, complete with burning in my eyes, breathing problems, sweats, swelling, and body pain. I don't remember being in that type of pain in all my life. But here's the catch: From what doctors told me, if they stop it too soon, you risk relapse. Stop it too late, you risk death. It's a delicate balance. When the time is right, doctors will give you steroids to calm the GVHD down. I laid in bed crying from the pain but refused to give in as I wanted the fight to rage on and save me. It was a mind over matter unlike anything I ever experienced before. Finally, weeks later, I suffered for as long as I could physically handle it and then said, "Give me the damn steroids— I'm good." Dr. Levis and his amazing Physician Assistant Jackie agreed.

Every guest or "caregiver" was a new way to pass the time. When my Papi was visiting, we played bingo and I cooked for him. Still, the days dragged on. I loved my caregivers, but I needed my space. They were slowing me down from my schedule. They each tried to baby me and tell me, "You already walked today. You need to take a break. You need to do this." I wanted to be in control. I'd had my survival schedule in place for ten months now and I knew the drill.

My caregivers came in and tried to tame me, to manage me. They each meant well but I wanted to do my routine of six walks a day. I wanted to write my stories. I wanted to research trials. I couldn't do all the things I had built around my survival with my caregivers. I found new ways to fill the time. We had fun. We made memories. But yet it was odd because I almost didn't know what to do since I was no longer alone. I found myself saying to each visitor/caregiver, "This is my writing time. This is cathartic for me. I am going to write for the next hour, so forgive me if I don't engage with you." The schedule I knew kept me alive while fully an in-patient at Hopkins worked, and I hated deviating from it.

At Hackerman, restaurants would often drop off food for patients in the community kitchen area and we would all sit and talk, play bingo or paint. I felt like I was at a senior home. We were all eager to see another person and talk about life before cancer, how we were initially misdiagnosed, how we missed our kids or grandkids, and what we would do different if we lived. We made friends with our hall mates, built a community, helped one another, laughed and cried for one another.

There were stories like the seventy-eight-year-old woman whose husband was misdiagnosed twice before doctors at Johns Hopkins diagnosed him with throat cancer. She thought her husband had bad breath. Other doctors said the same. Other patients shared their stories around a table as we played cards. Each patient and caregiver we met, each story of a misdiagnosis, was shared. Every single patient I met ended up at Johns Hopkins after being misdiagnosed or having their symptoms overlooked or minimized. It was baffling, while inspiring, hearing the stories that were shared and the lives that were impacted and how far patients came from for HOPE, ANSWERS and EXPERTISE offered at this world-renowned hospital.

I fully understood Johns Hopkins's policy to require patients undergoing this type of transplant or treatment to be a specific distance away. The hospital prides itself on successful outcomes. However, due to the financial toxicity of cancer, we were too broke to hire nurses to stay with me 24/7, and I barely had enough friends available to do so. In fact, my dad, who was battling his own health issues, came to be with me. While I love him, he was in NO condition to care for me. He couldn't push me in a wheelchair for help. In fact, some days I ended up pushing him. I cooked for him and somehow cared for him during his weeklong stay. I kept telling my dad, who worried he wasn't fit to care for me and be a caregiver, "Listen, I will have to overcome this too. I need you here. We can pretend you can care for me. They just want a human being to confirm being a caregiver. Right now, I need anyone with a pulse. I will save myself. Just please come stay with me."

Cesar couldn't miss work. My mom was taking care of Gabriel. My sister couldn't leave her kids. We had few options and no money. We faked it til' I made it. It worked. It doesn't mean it was right. The days wore on. I put up a mini-Christmas tree in my little "apartment." It wasn't like the Christmas tree I had put up at our house in Virginia with Gabriel, but it was enough to sit on the window sill and give me hope and a way to count down until my baby was back in my arms. I put tiny little ornaments on with pictures of our family. I needed to remind myself that I would be home for Christmas . . . even if by FaceTime, even if in my dreams.

Each visit back to the fifth-floor leukemia unit was a new hurdle. Setbacks and triumphs. Failed or successful blood transfusions, platelet donations, painful bone marrow biopsies, and sitting and waiting. The clock was ticking slowly. My emotions were wearing on me. I was getting tired, frustrated, and desperate to see Gabriel. Thanksgiving passed. Posts of family gatherings flooded social media and there I was, watching my counts, waiting to see my son, and waiting to see if I would live. It was surreal. I'm not a jealous person, but it was painful to watch the world go by as a spectator as my life hung in the balance.

One day as it got closer to Christmas, JoAnn came back to care for me. She insisted I get out and walk with my N95 mask away from the hospital for fresh air and perspective. I was nervous to be even a mile from the hospital. What if I spiked a fever? We hopped in the car to head a few miles away to grab lunch. The first song on the radio was *I'll Be Home for Christmas.* As the song played, we looked at each other, turned up the volume, and sang. As the we belted out the lyrics and they echoed throughout the car I was overcome by tears. I was overcome by emotion. I cried my eyes out.

Being home with Gabriel and Cesar in my arms did seem like a farfetched dream. I had lost all semblance of normalcy while I faced my mortality. It was like God was talking to me. HE knew what I was thinking. I wanted normalcy back. I wanted my life back. I wanted LIFE itself. I wanted to celebrate the birth of Jesus and my own rebirth and my life.

That next day at Johns Hopkins in the treatment room. I finally caved to my PA Jackie and to Dr. Levis. I made my case. "I have spent a year away from my son. I need a miracle. I need to be home for Christmas or I might die of a broken heart." They agreed, but only if I would agree to come back three times a week for follow-ups. I was scared to be far from help and my nurses and doctors but I rushed to my room. I almost skipped. I packed up all my things and like a Christmas miracle I was "home for Christmas".

But new challenges awaited.

CHAPTER 11

Faith and Fear

Spirituality is a big part of a pit crew.

For those who feel they don't need this chapter, hear me out. First, Spirituality doesn't necessarily mean religion. For me it did. It was one way for me to put my Armor of GOD on and ArmorUp for LIFE®. My faith is and was a part of my foundation. When you hit the LOWEST point in your life . . . believing in something BIGGER than YOURSELF is proven to be a successful form of coping. According to some studies, cancer patients who practice spiritual coping have higher survivor rates.

I can look back at some occasions in my fight that I did that very thing but with so much suffering. There was so much questioning. Faith has always been at the core of my foundation and impacted my daily decision making but I don't think I really "found my religion" and grew closer to GOD, connected and spoke to HIM, until I was staring death in the face. At the same time, I was also mad at HIM. Seeing so much suffering didn't make sense to me. I was witnessing it and I, too, was suffering. Physically, the chemo was breaking me down on every cellular cell. Mentally, I was losing it. Emotionally, I was distraught on so many levels. First, to watch my mom struggle to care for my son while worrying if her daughter would survive or not. Then to watch my son fall apart without me and not being able to understand what the hell was going on was another thorn in my flesh. And each day when my husband would walk into my room, I could see the exhaustion on his face and the fear in his eyes and I was heartbroken. How could MY GOD let something like this happen?

Ironically, it was also the time that I questioned where my GOD was with all *my* suffering and everyone else's suffering I was witnessing on the unit. I had so many questions. Why would He let me suffer in so much pain? Why would He let my son suffer and struggle away from me? Why were so many of us on the unit suffering? Why would He take my friend Ryan when his wife just had a baby and his kids needed him? Why . . . why . . . why?

I hated when the nurses would tell me, "Someone went 'home.'"

I would look at them and say with tears streaming down my face "Home? Home?"

They couldn't answer. I loved my Lord but I didn't want to go to any so-called home. What I truly wanted was to go to my own home in Virginia and into the arms of my son. My FAITH was on a collision course with FEAR and I couldn't get off the track.

I did my Christian/Catholic things. I punched the time card. I prayed the rosary, lighted my battery-operated candles, had the priest come by with holy water, prayed to my Angel Gabriel statue, and then I walked or shuffled to visit the big Jesus statue at Johns Hopkins daily, even if I had days I felt I could barely get there. I pleaded with Jesus, "Let me live. Spare my life and I will go out and serve others forever." I was deal-making. "God, I have a platform. I have a voice. I can reach people. Use me, speak to me, what else can I do? I need to see my son. Spare all of us. Let us all go home to our families." I would have conversations at this statue like, "Why are you letting so many people suffer?"

Yeah, I know this isn't the way you are supposed to pray, but it was MY prayer and how it was happening for me. I was running down the list of all the things I had done and wondering if there was something I was being punished for. I kept thinking, *I'm honest. I'm loyal, committed, love my family, I don't steal. . .* I was just that baffled.

Friends of mine in Texas and around the country reached out to local churches and friends of friends and asked them to come pray with me. However, even at that point, not all of them knew what to say or how to speak with me. I know, you probably think, *who needs a class to go in and pray with a patient.?* You can't go wrong with GOD, right? Well, you can when it comes to your delivery. I was in awe of what some people said, but it all came from a kind heart.

I was grateful for their time but couldn't wait for them to leave. They meant well, but their words were the last thing I wanted to hear. They stirred up more anxiety, and left me in a panic because, once they left, I was all alone in that room and some days it was total isolation. When I say isolation, I mean, no one could enter without an isolation gown on. No touching. No visitors. I never really had visitors because they were all in Texas. The few that I did have couldn't come, and I couldn't go. It was like being in a prison.

I wish I had the entire prayers and conversations written out, but here's what I remember. The key words in the last one are the winners. I was torn between my faith, my fear, and now my frustration.

"Dear Lord, please bring Loriana peace in her heart and help her cope and know when it's okay to surrender, and know it might be our time. When it's our time, then it's our time. We are ready for you."

In my head, I would be saying, "NOOOOOOO! What? It's not my time! It can't be my freakin' time. Speak for yourself! My family needs me. My husband needs his job. Clearly no one can take care of our son without panicking. My mom is having a mental breakdown. My sister's family is already overwhelmed. My dad and Jane have my dog and that's all I can handle. I don't have time to die, so no I'm not ready for you."

"Please, Lord, surround us with your arms, help us cope and when it's time to go HOME. We are ready to go home."

HOME? No Sir. No way am I READY to go home? Not HOME HOME? You have got to be kidding me. Everyone who died on this hall left their kids to grow up with just one parent when they went HOME. Yes, I wanted to go HOME, as in to MY house in Northern VA. Let's be clear on this. I can go HOME HOME and praise you when I'm 100, but I have work to do, memories to make, lives to impact and save through advocacy, a son to raise, a husband to love, parents to spend time with…. No thank you. Not today...let's talk in fifty years and we will be cool.

The HOME HOME also struck a chord with me because when patients did "check out" and went HOME HOME, as in "home to be with the Lord," it was devastating. To this day I cannot call my husband and say, "Hi honey, I'm on my way home from the store" or wherever I'm headed home from. I say, I'm headed back to the house.

Now to the best one yet. The kindest, sweetest older woman came to spend time with me. She stayed an hour. She prayed a rosary with me. She asked me about my family. She shared stories of hers. She looked on the wall and saw pictures of Gabriel and said, "You have one son?" I said "yes." She said, "Oh no honey, I have three. You need more. *You need a spare.* I lost my child in an accident and I'm thankful I had other kids so they have each other."

I sat up, and almost bit her head off and while sobbing I said, "I was trying to have a 'spare' when I ended up here with leukemia. So no, I don't have a spare. Stupid cancer robbed us of a 'spare.'"

I cried and kindly thanked the woman for her time and asked her to leave, and then all day I was NUTS. It pains me to this day that I haven't had that second child that we so desperately want. That our son asks for EVERY. SINGLE. DAY.

Instead, I turned to FaceTime and friends who knew me well and prayed with them. My friend Todd and his wife Valerie always prayed with me. So many others did as well. They chose each word carefully and knew what I could handle.

So, while I say spiritual counseling is a great way to cope, it needs to be the right fit. Despite all those fears, I did choose faith. On my terms, with what I could handle.

I know when my oncologist told me to "put my armor on" that I would be in this fight for the year. If I survived, then I needed the *ARMOR of GOD* to get me through it. I knew I needed prayer and a "pit crew" of prayer warriors to see me through, to pray with me and pray for me.

A cross-sectional study was done on 101 patients undergoing intravenous chemotherapy in an oncology outpatient center. The results from this study reinforced the notion that religious/spiritual coping is an important strategy for coping with cancer.

Why? Because religious people frequently present a greater capacity for coping with adverse circumstances in life. Another interesting finding from this study—80% of the patients expressed a desire to receive spiritual care and considered this as an important way to help cope with the disease. However, only 16% of the patients interviewed had received any type of spiritual care. Both the lack of professional training in spiritual care and the precedence that physical care takes over any other kind are reasons that this holds true, but also stand as proof that something needs to be changed. There are three ways that spirituality can and WILL improve your life:

1. Spiritual support groups help provide a sense of belonging and safety. Ask your hospital social worker or oncologist to connect you with a spiritual group in your hospital.
2. Studies have shown that spiritual people find ways to meet challenge with purpose, and bounce back and carry on.
3. Spiritual people make healthier choices—adhering to a particular spiritual tradition will encourage you to treat your body with kindness and avoid unhealthy behaviors.

One research study: https://www.scielo.br/scielo.php?script=sci_arttext&pid=S0104-11692013000200539 sought to investigate the use of religious/spiritual coping among people with cancer undergoing chemotherapy.

Having FAITH played a role daily in my survival, but there were four poignant moments I remember clearly:

1. *Returning to the hospital after finally seeing my then twenty-two-month-old after our first fifty-day separation*

   He ran away from me and didn't remember me. He walked past me like we had never met. That moment was more painful than the chemo that ran through it. I screamed, cried and asked "Why me?" I had one week with him. It took three days for him to let me connect and really hold him. On day seven, I had to say goodbye not knowing if it was the last time I would live to see him again. I cried and didn't know what to say. I looked at him hysterically crying and said, "Mommy's going to the store. I'll be right back," when "right back" could have meant forever. There was a 75% chance I wasn't going to live to see him again and that day would be my last time with him. I had to have FAITH I would beat the odds and come home to him.

   My husband took him from me and headed to the airport to take him back to Atlanta to live with my mom, and then returned to get me and take me to check back in for another round of hell. It was a dagger in my heart. I asked, "Why can't I see him each day?" My doctor said, "You have no immune system. His germs can kill you. You won't even have a chance to fight this battle. You can live in the short term, be with your son and let his germs potentially kill you, or look at the long term, Have FAITH that you will live and you will have him forever." That was the hardest thing I ever had to do.

2. *My sister, my angel, and MY HERO*

Nine months into treatment, when the doctors realized that the current treatment of high intensity chemo didn't knock down my cancer and instead it was coming back, they did a search for bone marrow donors. I couldn't believe the donor list is more than 70 percent Caucasian. They were having trouble finding a match for me. My sister was a perfect match, but she had a heart murmur so that wasn't a guarantee. She had to pass a week of rigorous tests. I remember sitting in the waiting room as she went through each test crying and praying for her to pass. It was so stressful. My life was in her hands and the condition of her health. I knew that once again I had to put FAITH over FEAR to get through this. I rejoiced when they said they would pass her because she was so fit that the murmur was okay. Praise the lord!

3. *Christmas in October*

Nine months into treatment, my cancer came back and I needed a bone marrow transplant. It was my only hope. They let me see Gabriel for one week before that transplant and I'll never forget the words from my oncologist and my psychologist.... "Go home and celebrate Christmas early. Decorate a tree. Make memories and take plenty of pictures so your son has that memory of you. There's no guarantee the transplant will work." I knew that first hand because I had lost friends post-transplant and I was terrified. So, my sister flew in to save my life and be my donor. But before we checked in—We went to

Walmart in mid-October, and in tears I scrambled looking for any tree that would light up so I could pretend it was Christmas so he could have one last memory of me if in case the transplant didn't take. There were so many struggles over the 100 days after the transplant. Victories and defeats. I was terrified. Putting my FAITH over FEAR helped me cope. I checked out Christmas Day as a Christmas MIRACLE. I put the Armor of GOD on each and every day. I made a promise to GOD that, if I lived, I would always show gratitude, help others, serve those in need, speak for those who no longer can, and celebrate Christmas early as a symbol of my gratitude.

4. *Every night, I walked the halls like clockwork.*

I needed sleep but was scared to sleep too long because I always questioned if I would wake back up. Many in my unit didn't. One night, at 2 AM, a man came to check his wife into the unit. She had an aggressive form of leukemia. But he said he was told that her heart wasn't strong enough to tolerate the chemo. They told him she had to go to cardiology FIRST and get her heart right and then go come back. He walked the halls sobbing and came up and asked, "why are you walking so late?" I told him that I walked each step for my son. Each step put me another step closer to seeing him. I told him I would pray with him as others had done with me. He told me he didn't believe in GOD. I said, "Then be a hopeful man and I will pray for you." We stood in the hall, cried, held hands and asked GOD for guidance, and the next day we turned to prayer warriors to help. It was a powerful moment of spirituality.

Humanity is the marker. We all are in this together and we all need to lift each other up.

CHAPTER 12

Identity Crisis Losses

E ven when you win, you lose. Pivot and find purpose.

You've heard the saying, "Life begins at the end of your comfort zone." I redefined it. I had a second chance at life and I was so uncomfortable that I became miserable. But try to complain about anything in your life after cancer or a crisis like the pandemic, and you will be sure to have someone say, "Oh, but you are alive! Be grateful."

Oh, I am! Trust me, from the minute my feet touch the floor I consider each day a gift. But understand that just because we won doesn't mean we haven't suffered loss. Most survivors do. It also doesn't mean we don't deserve quality of life, which in many cases comes with a trade-off and risk of a potential secondary cancer.

I lost nearly everything almost down to my soul, including my DNA. The very thing I worked hard to build and fought so hard not to lose, I lost anyway.

I LOST my identity.

- My chance to have my baby on Oct 11th
- My period and youth
- My son for my one-year fight
- My hair
- My ability to care for myself
- My strong immune system
- My strength
- My career
- My friendships—some friends walked away and didn't know what to say
- My DNA. Post-transplant, I now have my sister's DNA
- My identity—I was no longer the same person physically or mentally
- My fertility—chemo damages your reproductive organs
- My connection & intimacy with my husband
- My quality of life—the long-term effects of treatment leave you damaged

Then, one by one, I lost friends on the hall (Ryan and Paul, among others). The losses pile up. They change you. You will never be that person you once were. But to get through this, you have to mourn the loss of the person you once were and embrace who you are today and where you are today. *That. Is. Hard.*

Have HOPE. Have FAITH. Get HELP.

Your pivot will help lead to your passion but it doesn't happen overnight. I remember my darkest days. I've been there often. There *is* light at the end of the tunnel. If you are lost right now, pull strength from other survivors. We more than anyone know loss, isolation, depression, germ warfare, and going paycheck to paycheck, if there even was one.

I remember screaming at my husband one day during my daily meltdowns. I was angry he didn't understand me. My anxiety. My fears. The PTSD. The trauma. One hundred days after my bone marrow transplant, I was finally reunited with my son on Christmas Day. What was supposed to be a Christmas miracle turned out to be a nightmare because my baby boy looked right through me like he didn't know me. I felt lost and didn't know what to do with myself. I found myself in a mind and body I no longer recognized. I had a 25 percent chance of living another five years. I felt tormented.

Do I make resumes in case I live, or memories in case I die?

Even my own husband who saw me suffer didn't understand how much I changed. Why wouldn't I go to large events with him? Why did I refuse to take a train? Why did I fear death at every turn? One night he looked baffled by it all and I *lost* it! I began to scream and punch the walls. Cesar looked at me and I could see it in his eyes. He wanted to say, "Who are you? You are not the person I married." But instead he said, "Honey, I am so sorry. I feel like I don't know what to say anymore. I have to learn the new you."

I screamed, "How the FUCK can you know me, if *I* don't even know me?"

I was so lost.

The next day when my husband left for work, I officially cracked. I found out his company was restructuring and he needed to take a new position in Philadelphia. Even worse, I wasn't healthy enough to move. What? Another loss? You must be kidding me. How much shit could I physically handle?

I went from living my life in a successful on-air career to fighting for my life and then eventually wanting to take my own life. In my career as an Emmy Award-winning broadcast journalist, I had moderated political debates, interviewed presidents, unraveled the most complicated stories for viewers, and yet I couldn't cope with being alive. I began to pound on the wall separating our carriage home from our neighbor's. I was behaving like a lunatic. I was having a nervous breakdown. I was moments away from closing the garage and starting my car. I couldn't see a way up or way out.

I would sit and think, *If I do this, who will watch Gabriel while Cesar works twelve to fourteen-hour days? When will he go learn other extracurricular activities? Who will do homework with him?* It sounds strange after doctors and nurses had worked so hard to save me that I wanted to just check out permanently, but I didn't know what to do with myself. The stress of not knowing IF you are going to live and not knowing HOW to live is overwhelming. Adding to that stress was the financial toxicity of cancer, and the enormous pain in my heart of wanting another child.

Sadly, what happened to me (us) is not unusual for the cancer patients or those impacted by COVID, whether physically, emotionally, psychologically or financially. There is so much talk in the medical community, "We want more people to survive, and those who do have a better quality of life." Amen. Thankfully more people are surviving, but what systems do you have in place for us when we survive? Mentally, physically, emotionally, financially, professionally to help us reintegrate?

We are more than just a symbol QoL.

Measuring patient outcomes can't only mean we are breathing because often, if we are, we are still so very broken we don't know how to move on. There is **NO** reintegration program like the military offers to veterans returning home. No one follows you through the system to see how you are. Even convicts leaving prison have to check in with probation officers to track their progress and get them back into society to build them back up and put them back together—to live their lives. That's what we need—the WHOLE PATIENT APPROACH

There's no one to help your husband shift from caregiver to husband.

There was NOTHING. No strategic plan . . . just GOOD LUCK and *adios!* See you for your follow-ups and flare-ups of problems. But what about the rest of me that's broken? I was coping and cracking at the same time. The healthcare system is good at beating back death, but there is no one who gives you the tools you need for success.

It was one of the darkest days of my life.

But I also knew I had a bigger purpose and that I had PROMISED GOD that I would put HIS armor on and serve and help others if my life was spared. I would ArmorUp for LIFE®.

Depression from so much loss is something many are struggling with after managing COVID-19. I see it in their faces. I hear it in their stories. I worry about them. I was *one* of them. I'm still one of them on some days or some hours. It's another dark place I never want to revisit. But I do believe those struggling can and should turn to survivors like me for where and how we found our strength and light at the end of the tunnel, how we found the strength to rise from the ashes.

I tried each day not to feed the fears but the reality makes it tough. The limbo of waiting caused an enormous amount of anxiety. As a well-known quote says, "Fear, uncertainty and discomfort are your compass toward growth." They were for me. They can be for you.

What the system was lacking, I had to build on my own. I hope to one day, through funding with ArmorUp for LIFE®, help others build their crew or be the pit crew they desperately need through support and counseling. Please, wave the flag and ask for help. Build your pit crew again. Humble yourself and ask professional and personal friends for help. It's okay to do so. If you don't ask for it, how in the world will anyone know you need it?

TAKEAWAY

Humble yourself. Ask for help and delegate!

PTSD is real. Cancer-related PTSD is real. I'm still in treatment for it and so is my now eight-year-old son. We are veterans of a different war. Patient, caretaker, or loved one—no matter who you are or what type of cancer you face, loss is part of the journey. So are depression, anxiety, loneliness, scan-xiety, job losses and debt. For everyone the collateral damage is different. Recognize it. Don't deny it.

The good news is, there is an emerging field called Psycho-oncology, because the medical field is *finally* starting to understand the desperate need to treat the whole patient. *Psycho-oncology* is an interdisciplinary *field* at the intersection of physical, psychological, social, and behavioral aspects of the *cancer* experience for both patients and caregivers. While this represents a major step forward in terms of care for the whole patient, it doesn't mean patients or caregivers are getting the help that they need. Some cancers have more available help than others. It comes down to funding and support. That same support system will be desperately needed for those affected by COVID-19.

On the medical side, Dr. Levis is my HERO. He's one of the best and brightest. He is world renowned and I love him. But he needs support. He has no one helping him handle the psychological side of treatment. He shouldn't have to bear all our burdens. I've leaned on him for so much well beyond his scope of work. There was no sign of psycho-oncology in 2014, and even in 2020, it's not being applied like it should.

From my personal experience and that of others who have reached out to me, there is NO continuity of care except with your oncologist. No one follows you through the system. After the last drip of chemo and 100 days post bone marrow transplant, it's like, "Bye, good luck . . . see you at your appointments." Once we knew my blood counts showed I remained in remission we both were so thrilled! Yes, another small victory. I lived from blood draw to blood draw. I still do! He would smile and say, "Go make memories with your son." He knew the stats.

My response was always, "But what about the rest of me that is broken?" My mind and my body from head to toe had issues from the toxicity of the treatment. I needed a team of doctors, including neurologist, ophthalmologist, gastroenterologist, medical dermatologist, infectious disease doctor, immunologist, endocrinologist, psychologist, podiatrist and more to deal with the damage that had been done. Dr. Levis couldn't manage it alone.

Over the years I still look in the mirror and ask, "Who am I?" It was like the scene out of *Alice in Wonderland* where Alice asks, "Who in the world am I? Ah, that's the great puzzle." It *is* a great puzzle. I wish someone, some brilliant researcher, could make me feel whole again. I know what it feels like to be in good health, and being on the opposite end of that spectrum was uncomfortable. It was unfamiliar territory. Professionally it was like I was chasing a damn carrot that kept getting pushed back.

Many survivors struggle with PTSD. It haunts me to this day. Every decision I make is based on "what if something happens?" I worry about, "what if I die and don't see my son again?" I remember how much he struggled and continues to struggle. I don't like large crowds unless I'm speaking. When I am on stage, I'm happy. I don't like concerts. What if I get trampled? I'm scared of trains. What if they derail? I'm scared of icy/weather conditions. What if I crash?

Our son, Gabriel, continues treatment for PTSD. He's eight years old now. Every time I'm sick, he asks if it's cancer and if they are taking me away from him. Even recently when I got the flu, he laid next to me for days. He puts a washcloth on my forehead. He takes my temperature constantly. If I have bone pain and walk slowly, he asks if that means I'm aging faster and will die sooner. He panics when I'm late to get him at school.

Despite all of this loss, you can do this!

You just need the tools to navigate and a team to support you.

Medically

- Focus on the whole patient. The whole *you*. Push to see doctors for each issue from head to toe, mind and body.
- Ask for transportation help.

You have to be assertive and ASK for referrals to specialists to put the pieces back together and make you whole again. Don't just settle with "this is the new you" and not treat these issues. The new you needs help.

Patient compliance is a HUGE issue in the medical industry, but transportation is one reason we don't comply. We can't get there. We are too broke to afford alternate transportation and our spouses can't afford to take off of work. In many cases, patients who used time off to fight cancer or COVID likely won't ask for more time off for recovery. It's a decision that ultimately comes down to health insurance and finances. But they *need* that time to heal.

During treatment, the time when I really needed to be held, we were not allowed to sleep next to each other because of germs and risk of infection. Cesar slept on a pull-out couch and I was in my hospital bed. At times, I would try to hold his hand across the bed but my husband was so tired trying to care for me, fly back and forth to Atlanta to see our son, and hold down a demanding senior leadership job in the news industry that he would walk in my room each day, look at me, and pass out. Affection and intimacy weren't feasible or desirable. Your focus is survival. The problem is, once you get out and you are in recovery, you are so exhausted and broken by missing all the things you dreamed of doing, you can't afford to do them. You also learn one of the darkest secrets of cancer survivorship and marriage. The internal damage from the chemo makes sex painful for a long time. This is something only survivors talk about privately. It's actually one of the darkest secrets of cancer.

> Make sure at the very beginning of your battle, or your loved one's battle, that you ask for help psychologically.

This chapter is enough to send me over the edge. LOSS and its impact on survivors is so grossly overlooked that it's maddening to me.

I'm not dismissing the tragic loss we suffer when we lose someone to this ugly fight. They will forever be in my heart and I'll always fight to be a voice for them. I still get treatment to deal with the physical loss of those who can no longer fight.

> You are allowed to have high standards and want more. Don't let people make you feel like it's okay for everything else to suck because "hey, you made it." Let this pivot help find your passion. Set goals and go for it.

The old cliché "The new normal" sends chills down my spine.

We still want quality of life and that includes our mental health. It also includes our physical health. To the medical field, it's simply QoL, but it's not three letters that should easily be tossed around. In most cases you can't go back to doing what you loved; your hobbies have to shift. Your standards have to change. My doctor used to refer to other problems that circled around me as "petty torments" but really this was more like collateral damage. The loss was immeasurable.

Start Delegating

This is a good skill to learn while you are fighting anyway.

When you read my story on paper you wonder where the team of social workers was during and post-treatment. Even a non-trained lay person can read this brief description and see holes in the system. I was hospitalized for a year, separated from my then two-year-old son for an entire year except four brief visits where he didn't recognize me, a pregnancy was cancelled, and a seventy-year-old grandma was given guardianship to raise him alone.

No one told me what to tell him while he sobbed on Face-Time and asked, "How many more sleeps?" I could barely look at Gabriel because I couldn't tell him and didn't know my fate. During those four occasions when I *could* see him, after one week I had to give him back and I would cry hysterically. I would say, "I'm going to the store." To this day . . . he doesn't believe me when I say I'll be right back. I can't say the system failed me because there was no system in place to fail.

No one to help me navigate this crisis.

> If they can give a crisis team to someone in the military and teach that family how to prepare for separation and potential loss . . . then it can be done for cancer patients too.

I put together my own PIT CREW of psychologists to help. I even reached out to our FOX On-Air Contributor to help. But I was fortunate to have her on speed dial. Not everyone has that luxury. I had contacts far and wide and could fill the voids in my treatment but what broke my heart is that not everyone does.

ArmorUp for LIFE® is working to help educate the cancer community so it can understand this gap in treatment, so everyone has someone to help them psychologically from start to finish. When I say "finish," not after the last drip of chemo, but through survivorship because we all know that cancer doesn't end after you walk out those hospital doors. Even if you are in remission, the "petty torments" or "collateral damage" follow you for a lifetime.

Patient Navigation and a better overall experience are what building this "PIT CREW" is all about. For now, it is up to you to become your own HERO and your family to become YOUR HERO and ask for the help.

Professionally

This part of my recovery was and remains a real challenge.

What about the twenty-plus year career I had busted my ass building as a news anchor, a fitness/health reporter, and a brand? I was stuck in the middle of, "Am I going to live and what am I going to do now?" I was tired and needed to rest, but the terrified driven person inside said "rebuild, rebrand and make a new resume in case you live."

Given my PTSD, anxiety, inconsistent health problems, and constant medical appointments, there was no way I could go back to the demanding twelve to fifteen hour days of TV, much less in a new city, no matter how much I loved it. My body's immune system isn't programmed for that anymore.

I know I'm not alone. For those who do go back to work, they can't always hold down the same positions. Repurposing yourself isn't easy. You have to take into account who you are, what your position is, what skill set you still have, and what can you now do. That process can literally require a spreadsheet comparing job responsibilities and what you can or cannot do.

If more patients are surviving cancer, we better start planning on how to repurpose them in their existing careers or in new ones, or we are going to have millions who can no longer provide for themselves and a community dependent on help to survive.

One of my best friends called me and said, "I can't take away your cancer or pain but I can do what I know, and that will help you get back up."

It was the best gift I could ever ask for. This friend, Amy, has been my mentor and best friend through this entire struggle, along with others like my friends Janice Caprelian, Drex Earle, Jason Stanford, Natali Ceniza, Melissa Rauscher, Amanda De-Palma, and Kristine Illaria. I was so blessed that many of my friends came to my aid and coached me through these stressful years. They volunteered time and have become my mentors and heroes. Even today they are still there for me.

I was blessed to have a very distinguished contact list of who's who which included many CEOs. Sadly, what breaks my heart is not everyone does. I want to change that. *ArmorUp for LIFE®* wants to make this assistance part of its patient experience and platform, putting survivors back to work.

I made a list of my skills and then started looking for what could be done on my own time which allowed for health scares like shingles, doctor appointments, and avoiding COVID and other illnesses due to my compromised immune system and being a mom.

> Dig deep and reach out to friends and career coaches to find the common denominators of your new skills to determine what you can do and then do something with it.

For survivors, including victims of the COVID-19 recession, take a deep breath. You can *pivot* and find *purpose* and reinvent yourself. It starts with making a list. Write down all your skill sets. What can you do? What skills do you offer? Find the common denominators and start deciding your next career path. Be open that it might be in a different industry. Be open to change.

For me, I found that advocating and speaking give me purpose. Using my voice to make an impact on others is cathartic for me. It's therapy for me to know that my voice can make the path better for others and improve patient outcomes; for those not yet facing illness, my voice has the ability to sound the alarm and save lives. That gives me strength to wake up each day. Cesar and Gabriel do too. Given my health issues, I am not fully reliable for anything consistent, but I know I can be a voice and help others and that's the role I've chosen. I can do it on my time, around my health issues.

Lifestyle

The financial toxicity of cancer impacts you in every way including how you live your new life. Your perspective changes but so does your income. You want to go out and live your best life but your medical bills are piling up. After escaping death and surviving cancer, when you get out of the hospital you want to go do all the things you dreamed of doing. You want to go out and make memories and take steps to limit the stress in your life but you are too broke to do it.

ArmorUp for LIFE® hopes to one day fill that gap for patients because after all you go through, you deserve a family vacation or to mark one thing off your bucket list. When I got home and began focusing on working out beyond my hospital walks, I added in yoga and got back to my clean eating and green drinking, which included juicing raw veggies and drinking bone broth.

Then, the biggest thing of all, I PRIORITIZED my sleep.

Despite so much loss, I have been blessed with incredible gains.

Leukemia doesn't own me. It transformed me. It repurposed me.

CHAPTER 13

Gains

We often try to change our situation, but what we don't realize is that the situation we are in is meant to change us.

Leukemia certainly changed me. I never knew I could suffer with purpose, but I sure did.

For the first time in my life, I was forced to be still. It was time to re-center, time for prayer, time for introspection, time for gratitude. While I was on the go, walking my laps to avoid pneumonia and prepare for my fight, for the first time in my adult life I had a balanced schedule and I budgeted time to rest. Yes, it took leukemia to make me find pause in my life and schedule. For you, maybe it took COVID-19.

It didn't take me long to realize that if I lived, change needed to happen. Big change. I needed to slow down, prioritize my own well-being, give myself some grace, talk to God, reset my intentions, rest my goals, and adjust my dreams. Then, I could go forward stronger than before.

"The Lord will fight for you; you need only to be still." Exodus 14:14.

Post-Traumatic Growth (PTG)

One day as I shuffled through Johns Hopkins hooked up to chemo, I was given a button that said "Six-month SURVIVOR."

I quickly handed it back and said, "I'm not a survivor. I am still fighting."

They quickly corrected me. "Yes, you are a survivor from Day One."

We all are survivors of our own wars. Each and every day is a gift. Each day you are gaining a second chance at a new life. Make the most of it. Take your face out of your phone. Spend more quality time with your family. Make memories. You don't know what the future holds.

I can't talk about the loss without talking about how much I have gained from my cancer journey. Besides gaining weight (a side effect of all my meds) I have gained some things those outside the cancer community never truly understood until they experienced COVID-19: PERSPECTIVE.

I gained. . .

- LIFE. . . A second chance
- Resilience
- Strength
- Courage
- Gratitude
- A new lease on life and appreciation for each day
- A new perspective on life and what I will tolerate
- A desire to live my life to the fullest and live each day as if it's my last

- A greater sense or compassion for others
- An ability to say <u>NO</u> to negativity in my life and my circle of friends
- A bigger, more giving heart
- A hardened heart to those materialistic and full of petty complaints
- New friends with incredible hearts
- New opportunities to serve and help others
- A pit crew of friends/professionals to help me get back up
- A renewed faith in the kindness of strangers and the good in our world
- A renewed faith in my faith and my GOD

I touched on Post-Traumatic Growth in Chapter Six, but I think it is worth visiting outside of the context of my fight chapters. The Post-Traumatic Growth term was coined by Richard Tedeschi and Lawrence Calhoun to capture the idea of a positive psychological change that is experienced as a result of the struggle with highly challenging life circumstances or a traumatic event. The focus is when that traumatic event challenges our core beliefs and we find a new sense of growth.

Here is a list of what changes can often be seen as a result of PTG.

- Greater appreciation of life
- Improved relationships with others (the little things aren't so bothersome anymore)
- New possibilities in life—new purpose

---

https://www.apa.org/monitor/2016/11/growth-trauma

- Personal strength
- Spiritual change and development
- Creative growth
- Increased compassion

You might have traumatic events that pushed you through PTG. COVID-19 is forcing so many into and through some of this very growth. It wasn't planned for. The trauma and the anger might come first, but the growth will follow. Psychologists say that growth comes from us no longer being able to change a situation. This challenges us to change ourselves. The pandemic certainly fits into that criteria. You are being forced to restructure and rebuild like I did many years ago. You are now positioned to pursue and embrace those new opportunities.

I will point out that, while my heart has grown softer, and kinder for many, it hasn't for everyone. After staring death in the face, I think it's written all over my face when someone cries to me about something that I think is a "first-world problem" and ridiculous in the big picture of life. I can no longer relate and don't know how to respond.

I can't tell you how many times I have scrolled through social media or just listened to friends talk and thought to myself, *"Are they kidding me? Did they just cry because they couldn't get the beach house they wanted?" "Are they upset that their birthday party wasn't large enough?"* What usually comes to mind is . . . be blessed you had a birthday AND a party. Be blessed you woke up today and had another day.

Survivors . . . your perspective will change too.

I don't know if I ever took that much for granted, but I do know I was like many of us, living life like nothing was ever going to happen. I thought I was invincible and crying over ridiculous things. After cancer, I found myself telling my son what my Papi, who escaped communist Cuba, would tell me. "You can lose it all in an instant. Don't let greed and materialism become who you are."

My life as a news anchor and fitness/health reporter meant I did have an exciting lifestyle at times and had opportunities to attend high-end social events. But I tried to never take it for granted. I also had a lot of time to advocate for others and volunteer for some amazing charitable organizations. I loved my work. I loved those I helped and the people I met along the way.

> But I never really knew the true impact of the work I was doing until the tables turned and I was in need of the help I once gave.

I don't think I was truly in it each time I volunteered. It just sounded good, so I did it because I love to help. Now I understand the full impact of donation dollars and the lives that are changed and saved.

CHAPTER 14

Recovery

Cancer does not end after the last drip of chemo; the struggles and the fight just take new shape. You come out of this alive, grateful but very broken. While we are seeing more patient navigators in some areas of the cancer space, they are not everywhere and their work is limited to your current treatment. Once they set you free, you are on your own to navigate, yet the problems you will face can last a lifetime.

Survivorship programs are slowly taking shape. We are even seeing more well-known institutions add departments like "cardio-oncology" to monitor your heart long after the cancer is gone. The so-called "petty torments" of the treatment, which actually feel like a new hell, start to roar once you go home, but all that matters to everyone are your blood counts. The support you have from friends and the community start to fade because they think you are done and back to "normal."

I admit, as patients we can be guilty of feeding this problem with our doctors. We walk into our appointments with long lists of problems, but after sitting in the waiting room sweating and stressing about our white counts, once our doctors say, "Your counts are good," we breathe big sighs of relief. Good white counts indicate no sign of cancer. Suddenly our long lists of other issues take a back seat again, but they impact our quality of life and they must be addressed.

I felt guilty knowing that, just a few floors up, others were dying, so when I would respond with saying, "Amen, but I'm still depressed. What about my memory problems, or my heart issues and vision loss? What about my neuropathy? When I try to lie down and read books to my son, the bone pain in my feet is enough to make me cry. When I am out with my family, I can't stand long in one place because my feet go numb and burn. Oh, and my stomach issues—the GI issues? Oh, and how do I get this covered since we are broke?"

While they were my immediate problems, I knew others didn't even live to see the day to suffer through them. It's hard to look your doctor in the eyes and say this when he has patients upstairs who may not live to see tomorrow. But we as survivors have to look to our future. ArmorUp for LIFE® is hoping to continue advocating for more patient support and help build those pit crews, but we desperately need more research. That's what the *Leukemia and Lymphoma Society* is working on. Answers. We need more people to survive, and for those who do to have better quality of life.

There are nearly 17 million cancer survivors in the US, and reports say by 2026, there will be nearly 20 million survivors. Many of us can't go back to do what we are qualified and trained to do. We are broken, but the system forgets us. We are checked off with a big green check as a successful patient outcome and they move on.

I quickly learned I needed to build another "pit crew" for my "new norm" of needs and struggles. It's like having a new car, but no instructions on how to put it into gear.

CHAPTER 15

The Cost of Winning

From Milestone to Madness

Orange pumpkins sat on the front porch, spice scent filled the crisp air, and fall was in full swing, but it was time to put our Christmas tree up. It's October! As Gabriel says every October 29, it's Halloween on the outside and Christmas on the inside! We love it!

We aren't early. We are right on time. The Christmas in October tradition started when my oncology team sent me home to see Gabriel before my bone marrow transplant. My leukemia had come back. We didn't know if I would survive the transplant. They told me, "Go home, put up your tree and take pictures with your son so that he has memories of you." That day the reality that I could die finally hit home with what I was dealing with.

Each year we honor that tradition. It grounds us. Reminds us of the reason for the season. It unites us that memories and life trump material gifts any day. But on the fifth anniversary, our friends suggested we change it up. Hold a tree-lighting ceremony and have friends come join us to decorate the tree. I hesitated. It wasn't the original tradition. I like routine.

But five years was a HUGE deal in the AML leukemia world. Remember, there was a 25 percent chance I would live to see Gabriel turn seven. The five-year marker is a milestone as far as patient outcomes (not for life insurance—I still can't get life insurance). We couldn't financially pull off the vacation, but something kept me from a BIG party.

I may have my flashy TV background but something about the smell of success with being cancer-free made my heart ache for all those who couldn't say the same thing. I never wanted to appear boasting, so I always would quietly celebrate my success of slaying leukemia. I was raised to never brag about your success, but just enjoy it while you have it. Perhaps it came from my Papi who fled communist Cuba after losing it all. He always said, "Enjoy the moment, and enjoy what you have because you never know if you might lose it." I thought I had already lost it. What else could possibly go wrong after five years of hell trying to get back up?

Two days before the party I went for a diagnostic mammogram and ultrasound to follow up on some swollen lymph nodes doctors had been monitoring for a year. Two months prior, I had seen a cardiologist for chest pains. He cleared me after thirty days of monitoring as being "unknown pain" or "stress-related." My appointment was at 1:00 PM in Baltimore. I figured by 2:00 PM I would be driving home, and by 4:15 I'd be back in PA. I mean, I think I paid my dues and then some when it comes to fighting cancer. It should have been easy sailing for me. I'm an advocate now, not a fighter. Been there. Done that.

But after the mammogram I was sent back out into the waiting room and waited and waited and waited. Women came and left. Some sat quietly, others made small talk and exchanged a few laughs. But one by one, they left. They called me back for a repeat mammogram of an area. Then I was sent back into the waiting room. Then they called me back to get the ultrasound to look at my lymph nodes. Then back out to the waiting room. Four-thirty rolled around. I was still there. I knew it was much more than my anxiety talking when I said, something wasn't right.

The tech came and said, "The doctor wants to see you in her office."

I knew it. No one needed to say it. I had cancer. I know how this works. I walked in; the doctor sat quietly, almost trying to find the right words. I had to help her.

I saved her. "It's okay. Say it, I have cancer, right? If you aren't going to take my son away for a year, if you aren't going to tell me I have a 25-percent chance of survival, then just tell me. Say it like it is and let me go home and get appointments lined up."

She looked at me and said, "Yes, I think you have breast cancer and I'm so sorry. I looked at your history and you have been through so much already. This isn't fair, but let's just get a biopsy and get this confirmed. There's a 75 percent chance it is not right."

"I like the sound of that. I had been living in a world of 75 percent chance that I would die. This diagnosis sounds so promising. It's all perspective!" I said to her.

Strangely, our party was the next day. It just seemed hard to celebrate my fifth re-birth and dance the night away to being cancer-free with a scheduled biopsy just days away and hanging over my head. But I have had scares before and skated by. I wanted to believe, in my heart, I would be fine. We had a house full of friends and celebrated. Plus, everyone always says, "Don't think about the worst-case scenario, think positive." That drives me crazy, BTW . . . I lived in the worst-case scenario. It's easy to let your mind go there.

Halloween Day was the first available biopsy. "Fine. I'll be there," I said, "But you better get me out of there by 11:00 AM so I can make it to Gabriel's school to volunteer by 1:00 PM. I promised him I would be there. Cancer, or the risk of it, will not steal another moment of my time with this boy of mine."

Cesar took me. I sat numbly in that chair with tears rolling down my eyes as I flashed back to everything I had already overcome. The doctor kept saying, "Are you okay? You aren't saying a word."

I would repeat to him, "This hurts, but it is no comparison to a bone-marrow biopsy. What hurts more is the fear, the fear of hearing that word again."

I made it to Gabriel's school. Somehow, I was able to smile through the pain. I decorated cookies with the class with an ice pack in my bra. I was determined not to let cancer overshadow the gift of time with my son.

Halloween night, I went trick-or-treating with Gabriel with another ice-pack and skipped through the streets almost in denial of the reality I could soon be facing. I wanted to believe this was all a bad dream. I was in so much pain, but I wouldn't dare let Gabriel know. I had made a living out of putting on a smile for my audience and that night would be no different.

I let Gabriel go well past his bedtime. Why not? It was a special night, after all. We were making memories. Another night that was a gift. As the night wound down, Gabriel saw the tape and marks on my right breast through my shirt. His face dropped. He asked if I was okay and if he could kiss my boo-boo. I explained that doctors just had to put a little pin in a bump on my breast. He insisted he wanted to touch the bump. He insisted he could make it go away with a mosquito spray and a little pressure on it. I could see the wheels of worry spin in his little head. I assured him Mommy was doing so well she would be heading to Chicago the very next day to speak to an amazing fundraiser to raise money for the very cancer she fought.

I got to the gate early that next day. To me, early is on time. After leukemia, I don't like to rush through life anymore. I don't like stress. I don't like to rush. I pulled up a chair near my gate, posted on Facebook how wonderful it is to be me, early at my gate, relaxed, heading to speak to an amazing crowd in Chicago and help others who walked the path I walked. I had finally arrived—sort of. I mean, I was living out my dream of helping others. Back at doing what I loved. And then the phone rang. It had a 410 area code. That meant Baltimore. My stomach always sinks when I see that area code. It makes me think of bad news from my oncologist calling to say I need to come back to the hospital.

I answered, "Hello."

"Hi, Loriana. This is Dr. DiCarlo. Is this an okay time to talk?"

"Yes, depending on what you have to say." I said with a nervous laugh.

"I'm sorry, but I wanted to let you know that you . . . you . . . you have cancer. Breast cancer. The biopsy came back positive."

I was shocked. The room stood still. I was numb. "Uhhh . . . okay. What do I do next? Where do I go? "

Dr. DiCarlo said, "I want you to call this number. This is the Johns Hopkins Breast Cancer Surgery Center. Tell them you spoke to me and that you need to see an oncologist."

While courteous and transparent, I was shocked at the process. In disbelief at how the system worked. At that very moment, it failed me. I had cancer. I needed someone to be there with me. Where was my navigator? What I wanted to hear was someone on the line with Dr. DiCarlo to say, "Hi Mrs. Hernandez-Aldama, I'm a patient-advocate or nurse navigator. I am on the phone with you and I will be here with you throughout this process. I am so sorry, but we will be with you each step of the way."

Instead, I hung up. Then I called the number all alone and said, "Hi, I have breast cancer. I don't know what to do. I was told to call this number and you would give me an appointment. Do I need to go somewhere or report in to someone?"

You see, with leukemia, I had to say goodbye to Gabriel and was rushed to the hospital. I had no idea what to expect and no one was there to help me, either. The receptionist said, "I'm sorry, but I don't see these results in the system. Are you sure you heard correctly?"

I stood there with the room spinning at the gate trying to decide. Should I just hang up and call Cesar, or should I try to convince this woman on the other end of the line that yes, I had cancer and I needed an appointment? She gave me an appointment for November 13th. Twelve (yes, twelve) days away. Wow. I didn't understand the lack of urgency. The loud intercom announcements were drowned out by my silent screams in my head. A bizarre numbness went over my body. I called Cesar much like I had to do the last two times I had to utter the C word. "Honey. Honey . . . I have cancer. I have cancerrrrrr AGAIN. What do I do? Do I go to Chicago?"

There was some part of me that felt like the warrior, the giver, the cheerleader inside of me needed to stand tall and get my ass on that plane and help others. However, the other half of me felt like this was eerily similar to before and that I *needed* to be home hugging my boys. I needed to just look at them and believe I was going to be okay.

Cesar said, "You aren't going. You need to come home. You need to process this." But my best friend Janice was halfway to Chicago to meet me. Was I supposed to just leave her stranded?

I left her stranded. Cesar picked me up. I left my car at the airport. He brought me home in tears. I knew, at that moment, I was just where I needed to be, and yet I felt guilty for leaving Janice and an entire audience at a cancer gala with no speaker. I've never not shown up for something. I'm a human doer and I just couldn't do what I usually do.

As we drove home, I felt like this was some cruel joke. I mean WTF, haven't I paid enough dues to society? Wasn't being separated from my son for a year and facing a 25-percent chance of survival enough to give me a lifetime of happiness and no worries? Wasn't there a trauma timecard we punched, and if so hadn't I met my limit?

That night Gabriel slept in my arms. He had no idea why I clung so tightly to him. Why should I tell him now? What benefit would it be to upset my sweet boy with the world of unknowns until I knew a game plan? That night, I sat numb in the bed with my world spinning around me. It was then I realized, saving my life came with a price.

And so there you have it. The most unexpected gift to celebrate being cancer-free . . . a secondary cancer. The trade-off, my doctors say, likely from the full-body radiation used to save my life.

Here we go again.

This time during COVID-19.

Thank GOD I prepared.

Thank GOD I'm ready.

I had a double mastectomy in January of 2020. It didn't go as planned. I was readmitted twice and spent weeks in the hospital during COVID. I faced three more infections and then had five months of home healthcare so nurses could "pack" my wound, the hole left in my breast. My husband ultimately had to be trained to do it for me.

I found more voids in the healthcare system. A system operating silo despite patients not healing in silos. I built another pit crew. I advocated. I pushed for answers. My message of the 3Ps gained an unofficial 4th P . . . PAIN IN THE ASS . . . to connect the dots and my healthcare providers to save my own life.

- I refused to accept the advice of my breast-cancer oncologist who insisted I only needed a lumpectomy, a decision he made *without* contacting my leukemia oncologist at the very same institution. A lumpectomy would have meant twenty days of radiation. In fact, he seemed annoyed that I would want to contact the very doctor who saved my life to help affirm his suggestion. Thankfully, after pushing to get in with my leukemia oncologist I found out that the full-body radiation I had received to save my life with my bone-marrow transplant meant I was not a candidate for a lumpectomy. Why did it take me connecting the dots to find this out? What happened to the whole patient approach? I became my own hero. AGAIN.

- My leukemia oncologist also insisted I get a double mastectomy because he said, "You simply don't know if there will be more." There was. As it turned out, the test results on both breasts removed from surgery revealed that I had not just one cancerous tumor but TWO!

- I ended up paving the way to get readmitted after going home from surgery by contacting my infectious disease teams at one institution to contact the other institution to readmit me. This came after a resident on-call dismissed my pain telling me, "Drink coffee; it's a diuretic," or "Stomach pain is not the reason to call the resident on-call at midnight."

- One long surgery, two re-admissions to the hospital for infections, five months of home health care to pack my wounds, delayed healing, and COVID-19 putting the world in a time out while my treatment went on hold.

I survived . . . AGAIN. Life is a trade-off.

What Gave Me Life . . . Might Ultimately Take it One Day

I learned that, when they gave me my sister's bone marrow and her DNA, they gave me her genetic marker which spun out of control. That marker is called CHIP, or "clonal hematopoiesis (generation of blood) of indeterminate potential," an autoimmune disease/cancer predisposition disease. It means that there was a subset of cells produced in my bone marrow that have mutated and will ultimately cause problems for me the rest of my life, however long that shall be. My doctor believes it may have happened when her marrow was transferred into me and put a lot of stress on me.

In the words of my doctor, "If I knew today what I didn't know the day of your bone-marrow transplant, I would have never given you your sister's marrow. She carries the CHIP mutation and now we know why you have suffered so much. You have been validated. Your pain now makes sense. Science is our marker (humanity is too), and we will look for science to advance faster than the disease will impact your life."

The truth is, my sister was my only hope of survival. The donor registry at the time was 70 percent white and I'm mixed race with Cuban and Italian roots. They had no other donors. My sister Lisa gave me hope. My sister gave my son his mother back.

In the words of Dr. Levis, "Your sister bought you time."

When I heard those words as I sat in his office during COVID-19, alone with no one at my side to help me process this, I looked at him and said, "I need to take my mask off so I can cry." My heart sank. "How much time?"

"I hope it is for a long time."

What I have learned from Dr. Levis is this disease means I am operating at fight or flight full time, 24/7, and my body is highly inflamed. There is no cure. The only way to get rid of it would be another transplant, which would carry a very low chance of survival. Dr. Levis once again closed this latest appointment with, "Go make memories and live life very carefully. Very carefully. Avoid all stress. Avoid inflammation-causing behaviors. Avoid surgeries.

Despite the odds, I am once again surviving.

It is up to me to own this disease and do my part to meet the medicine halfway. Surviving is my job. Anything that brings inflammation to my life will be out. Just like before. That won't change. Unhealthy food. Out. Toxic relationships and circumstances. Out. Lack of sleep. Out.

I will thrive and embrace the life I inherited. The DNA that is now mine.

I hope you embrace yours.

Remember . . . .

Life is a trade-off for all of us. Make the most of it.
Start preparing. Start living. Start resting. Stop stressing.
You have the chance today to "Become your own HERO."
I'm either your coach or your cautionary tale.
The choice is yours.
#ArmorUpforLIFE®

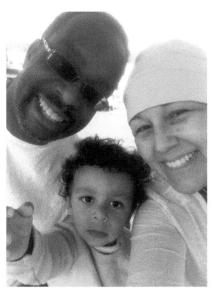

The Tool-Kit

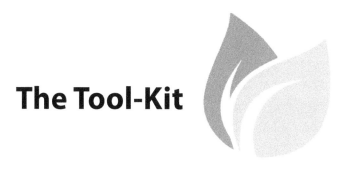

The tools you need to be an equal partner in your own success!

YOU the Patient

I'm sorry. I'm sorry your world has been flipped upside down. Getting a cancer diagnosis is so beyond difficult to process. The diagnosis sucks. It does. You are allowed to say that. I'm here to tell you that it's okay to be upset, it's okay to get worried, it's okay to get angry. You are *allowed* to put up your middle finger to the world and ask, "why me?" You don't have to put on a front to everyone. But once it sinks in that you do have cancer, and after you cry and yell and get pissed, let's get to work. We don't have time to waste. It's time to put your head before your heart and focus on the prize of winning and getting home to your family.

I'm not saying put your emotions on hold ALL the time, but you are embarking on such an emotional roller-coaster ride that if you don't put your emotions on hold from time to time to reflect, regroup, and focus on your game plan and setting goals, then it is easy to let depression, negativity, and thoughts of "what IFs" take over and you will lose your strength.

Whatever your job was, however important you feel you were BEFORE cancer, whatever image you have to uphold, however many projects you have due, deadlines to make, let it all go . . . none of that matters. WE ARE ALL ONE NOW.

Your Job Now is SURVIVING

Here's the problem:

Few people in your circle really know how to speak with you and help you. They mean well but they don't always say or do the right things. And once your diagnosis is public, EVERYONE you know becomes either an expert or has a story to tell about his/her connection to cancer and many of those stories will terrify you.

Those stories matter. The lives matter. They are coming from a good heart, but you can ask for everyone to hold tight on those conversations like . . .

"I know what you are going through, my mom died before transplant. She died when I was young and I grew up without my mom."

NOTE to friend—STOP—please keep this one to yourself.

I politely listened and then went into the hysteria of what would happen if I died. OMG! What if I don't make it to transplant? OMG, what if my son grows up without me?

The OMG's and What IF's went into overdrive and my stress went through the roof. I wanted to say. . . "HOLY SHIT—PUT A FILTER ON BEFORE YOU SPEAK," but I knew they meant well and didn't know how to say it kindly, so I share it on social media and made one group ask.

TAKEAWAY

Don't let these comments send you into a tailspin. Everyone will group all cancers into one lump. They are not. There are so many different cancers, different mutations, different factors that play a role. This will drive you crazy if you don't put this into perspective.

First, before you lump yourself into one group (*Caregivers remind your patient this on a regular basis too).

- How old was their mom?
- What year was she diagnosed?
- What treatment was available?
- Was she fit?
- Did she have other health issues (co-morbidities)?
- How much support did she have?
- How much stress was surrounding her?

ALL of this plays a role. We are all different.

How you respond, and the support from the pit crew you build (more on the pit crew in just a moment!) and surround yourself with, will help you and your family get through it.

Get a Plan

Take a deep breath, collect your thoughts, then get a plan. Sit alone with your family and cry. It's okay. You need to cry. Then get a game plan. What is the best plan to move forward? Do you have time for a second opinion, or do you need to get started on treatment immediately?

In my case, I had Acute Myeloid Leukemia (AML) and the mutation and type of subset I had meant it was urgent. I needed chemo running through my veins IMMEDIATELY. I didn't have time for a visit to Atlanta to see my parents and cry and just let it process. I boarded a plane alone to Johns Hopkins with my eyes set on the prize—winning. I got my plan, put my head before my heart, and went with what was best for my survival. I didn't have time to wait.

But remember, there are so many types of cancers, and within those cancers there are subsets and mutations. Breast cancer planning was so much different than AML leukemia planning. With blood cancer like AML you need treatment immediately. Every day is crucial. With breast cancer, I learned that you spend weeks and weeks just "chasing scans." Perhaps a bone scan to see if it has spread to other parts of your body. A CT scan to see if it has spread. There is scan after scan after scan.

The plan is that they only want to do surgery one time. If it's a lumpectomy where only the tumor and a specific area around the tumor are cut out, that often requires twenty days of radiation. A double mastectomy, which is what I had, did not require the setup of radiation. That's why it was best for me because my leukemia treatment had required full-body radiation and I was prohibited from having more. So, with breast cancer, be prepared to wait for appointment after appointment. You will go to sleep worried each night about waiting to remove the cancer.

Everyone is Different

Let me repeat this. We are all different. We show up to the fight differently We face different challenges. Age, fitness level, other conditions like diabetes, high blood pressure, obesity—they all play a role in how you "ArmorUp for LIFE®," the type of treatment you might receive and how aggressively you can be treated. You may have time to get other opinions and then develop a proper course of action. You may be able to do further testing.

Delegate

Assign your spouse, family member or friend to make calls for you and allow you to listen in.

Trust me when I say your mind will be racing with so much that you may not remember the full conversation about the types of treatment options. My husband thrives in crisis management, so he was the best person for me, but think of who you trust, and who can stay grounded and calm to make calls with you and for you. This person should be a good notetaker and not someone who panics easily.

Research

Call the organizations associated with your type of cancer and get information. After I called my family, my next call was to the Leukemia & Lymphoma Society. My husband had to make the call because my mind was too clouded to comprehend and remember what I heard, but LLS helped steer the ship for us. They gave us some options. They told my husband the treatment can be lengthy for leukemia. They were incredible with their help. There are other great organizations, large and small, making an impact. Some are more research-focused, and others are more patient-focused, but we are all in this together. Curing one cancer can, as I learned, put you in the land of another cancer, which is another reason we should help one another. Sometimes organizations also operate in silos and stay in their lanes, but the truth is research for one cancer has been found to help another cancer.

In addition to LLS and ArmorUp for LIFE® there are other great organizations. Reach out to them. Reach out to us. Let someone direct and guide you through this process. It isn't easy and we are STRONGER TOGETHER.

AACR - American Association for Cancer Research
American Cancer Society
Susan G Komen Foundation

Do Tell . . .

Set boundaries and communicate. I can't tell you how to handle the toughest moment of your life. It really is so personal to each and every one of us. So many factors are at play as to whether to share with family, friends or employer, and how to do so. I'm not saying to shout it from the mountaintop like I did all over social media, but I will say that I wholeheartedly believe my friends and supporters, my "pit crew," helped me cast a wide net for any help I asked for and any needs I had. I had so many friends on my hall who chose to tell no one and suffer in silence and fight alone. It broke my heart. I felt like they were ashamed.

Reach Out

You can't get help if you don't tell anyone you need it. I encourage you to open up and share your story. You will be in awe of the kindness in your community and you might save someone's life in the process when they hear your story. I also understand the tough decision this can be. especially if you fear how this might impact your career, your spouse's career, or your business. But I wholeheartedly believe that what you lose, you will gain in some other way. There is so much kindness in this world that good will somehow come out of this.

For business owners, I understand you might worry, "what if our customers think we aren't operating or we are not operating properly because I'm not there?" Can you assign someone to take over? Can you put an honest note on social media and explain that, yes you are operating and business is running as usual with someone else in charge?

For spouses or parents of those affected by cancer, I also understand this concern. My husband was so worried that his management would think he wasn't fully in the game that he over-compensated and worked non-stop.

ArmorUp for LIFE® will be happy to help you find an advisor to help you navigate this part of the process.

Communication Strategy

Decide how you are going to tell everyone and how much. Decide *who* will be the point of contact, *who* will be reaching out to friends, and be upfront with everyone about what you prefer.

For me, I took charge on many fronts, with the help of my amazing husband & rock, Cesar, at my side. We decided on what I would put out on social media and what he would handle each day.

My husband would take many calls for me because I was simply tired or so busy walking that I didn't want to talk. But when I was ready on some days, I would ask him who had called, and I saved all my return calls for my power walks. I would put on my Bluetooth, store all the numbers in my phone, and start walking. They kept me busy, and I didn't focus on how tired I was!

Be Honest and Transparent

You or your lead communicator needs to communicate what you need and how to help you.

We each have different needs. Be upfront. Ask for specific items.

Many people will rush to your aid with a kind heart and wanting to help. Let them. However, set boundaries because sometimes they say things that will upset you. So, let them know what you are willing to discuss but don't know how to. Others will retract and pull away from your life and leave you baffled. Don't be offended. These people who disappear don't know how to handle cancer, they don't know what to say to you, they don't know what kind of conversation to have, and they are scared. Others pull away because it is just too much for them. The good news is that, while some pull away, there will be angels who come into your life. You will gain so much more than you will lose.

What YOU the Patient Needs to Know

Your relationships will be strained. The stakes are high. The stress is insurmountable. The patience is low. Your relationships will be tested. Your strength will be challenged. Your memory will be impacted because it is simply so much to handle. Add to that, the effect of chemo impacting the brain. It's going to be . . . HARD.

Daily Tips

If you are hospitalized for your cancer treatment like I was, then you might have what's called "rounds" at your hospital. It's the process in which doctors make the rounds to each room to assess how the last twenty-four hours were and what the next twenty-four hours will look like.

I asked so many questions. They seemed to save me for last, but my doctor always praised me for pushing them for answers. They might be brilliant, and they may save so many lives but I wanted to be in their heads about "why this course of treatment over that one," etc.

- Create a daily journal with your questions and concerns. If you are in-patient like I was, I had a daily log of rounds when doctors came in and analyzed my case and my day-to-day blood counts.
- *Ask questions.* Tell your doctor(s) to slow down and repeat things. It's okay to say, "Can you give me an analogy and help me understand this in lay terms?" My doctor used to always give me analogies using the "queen bee" to relate to the T cells etc. Tell your doctor to come back and break down exactly what he or she said and what the next steps are. What are the pros and cons for today and for the long-term?
- *Look ahead.* Ask your doctor(s) what this means for tomorrow's strategy. What does all this mean for our "long-term strategy?" How will this impact the overall outcome? Think about what are you willing to do for survival versus for quality of life. You are not asking for too much to want both. Yes . . . ask for it and find out the next steps.

YOU the Caregiver/Family Member/Friend/ Co-worker

One of the biggest challenges I hear from caregivers is that they don't have time to mourn and process the tragic situation swirling around them. They are thrown straight into superhero mode. My husband always felt he had to be strong, since I was weak. Caretakers, know that you are so overlooked. You are appreciated.

Relationships—Know This

Your patience is low. Your relationship will be tested. Your strength will be challenged. You don't have time to reflect because you are doing so much for your loved one, but remember you have to prioritize YOU to have energy to care for your loved one.

- *Make time for yourself.*
  Just like the saying goes when you travel, "Put the oxygen mask on yourself first, then put one on your dependents." If you aren't healthy, you can't care for your family member. I know it is hard to take a break, to go on a walk, but you have to *re*charge so you can be *in* charge.

- *Take notes.*
  Be ready, because you will be overwhelmed.

- *Do your homework and don't be afraid to question decisions being made.*
  Even at world-renowned facilities like Johns Hopkins, doctors want you to ask questions, and to get involved.

- *Ask for help.*
  Be transparent about what you are struggling with, ask friends to give you a break. Ask family and friends for what you need.

- *Talk to a social worker on a regular basis.*
  It's okay to cry and then back to the business of caring for your loved one.

- *Continue the therapy after the treatment is over.*

  It will all hit you and you will need help processing what just happened.

Maybe the transplant or surgery "worked," but the fight doesn't end overnight. It is a long process and a lot of "collateral damage" that we as patients face. Don't let your help fade.

Here's a short list of many potential side effects of chemo and a cancer battle.

- Fatigue
- Depression
- Anxiety
- Anger/meltdowns
- Difficulty with focused thinking (chemo brain)
- Vision problems
- Early menopause
- Heart problems (chemo is fed through the heart)
- Reduced lung capacity
- Kidney & urinary problems
- Nerve problems, such as numbness and tingling
- Bone and joint problems
- Muscle weakness
- Secondary cancers

Ten Things NOT to Say to a Cancer Patient

1. Don't say, "Call if you need anything," because I have too much pride to ask. Just pick something and tell me

you are going to do it. See the list in the YOU the FRIEND section.

2. Don't text and say, "How do you feel?" That is really a loaded question. How long do you have? Texting me with "Thinking of you!" makes my day because then I won't feel obligated to engage in long conversations about how I am feeling because it is complicated and easier in a group message.

3. Don't say, "I know what you are going through, I lost my ____ to leukemia (insert cancer type here)." Please, while I am sorry you lost someone to cancer or faced something similar, now is NOT the time to share it with me. I can't emotionally process it but please know I care. Again, not all cancers manifest the same and we all show up different to this fight. Please don't start the wheels of death turning in my head. I need to keep my thoughts on winning.

4. Don't say NOTHING. Please don't disappear on me because you don't know what to say. Ask me what to say? Tell me you are new to this and not sure how to comfort me. So many friends disappeared on me and it broke my heart. I remember sitting up at night crying myself to sleep feeling so abandoned by people I loved so much.

5. OMG for the love of $%^& do NOT say, "Everything happens for a reason!" It doesn't. If it does, right now I can't look that far ahead to believe it.

6. Don't say, "You'll be fine!" My answer always was, "How the hell do you know? Ten people before you called just told me about friends or family members who died.

255

My doctor just told me I might die. Friends on my hall died. Do you have a crystal ball?" YES, I realize . . . I can also survive and I WILL and I DID!

7. I know "Stay strong" is a big one and I still believe I needed to "Stay Strong". I used to always say to my husband, "WTF does that mean? Strong is so subjective. How about telling me to, "ArmorUp for LIFE® and stay moving so you can be strong enough to meet the medicine halfway."

8. Don't say, "At least you look SKINNY." We don't want to be skinny; it's a side effect of all the vomiting and nausea. Reminding us how we look is not a compliment, no matter how you intended it.

9. Don't ask, "Have they told you your prognosis?" It's cancer. It sucks. When we are ready to share with you, we will. Perhaps ask, what the treatment plan is and what are the side effects we might experience.

10. Don't compare by saying, "I know how you feel." Even if you faced cancer, you can't know how I feel.

YOU The Medical Team

You are healers. You are heroes. We are thankful for you.

But please listen to us. Hear our cries. Listen to our concerns. Feel our pain.

Treat the whole patient, not just the one issue.

The healthcare system works in silos, but we don't heal in silos.

Don't discount our problems. Know we are whole patients with real-life problems.

I can't tell you how many times I had to push for my medical team to reach out to my other doctors, or that I had to personally connect them. My message might be PREPARE, PRESENT, PREVAIL, but my fourth and unofficial P is PAIN IN THE ASS. It's the only reason I truly believe I'm alive. Well, that plus the incredible heroes like Dr. Levis and my team of nurses who treated me.

Please don't dismiss our symptoms. Look at the whole picture. I was in awe of the countless times my own issues were dismissed. In isolation, they may not have been big issues, but combined with my history, I needed help and didn't always get it, from one doctor on-call telling me to "drink coffee" for pitted edema after healing complications post double mastectomy, to another telling me that "stomach pain is not a reason to call your on-call resident." I was in awe of many interactions I had when I later found out I was on my second infection post-surgery and needed an aspiration of fluid from my breast. The list of stories and experiences is long.

I often say, "We need to meet the medicine halfway, but YOU the medical team also have to meet us halfway."

Recipes—Elevate Your Plate for "Clean Eating"

Elevating your plate doesn't mean taking the flavor out; it's about putting the nutrients in. Whether you are a patient going through treatment or someone just trying to ArmorUp for LIFE® and get your body prepared for illness and to fight, I highly recommend giving these recipes a try.

These recipes are for EVERYONE, but if you are a cancer patient or survivor, they are especially for you (or for you to send to friends to make for you and send to you!).

When I had leukemia, I didn't have much of an appetite, but I knew I needed to eat. The problem was there was NO way I was going to drink the disgusting sugar-filled, processed protein shakes in the pantry on the unit, nor would I eat the hospital food which had fruit and ice cream "smoothies" for those days when you couldn't chew. I knew that sugar feeds cancer and I already had cancer. I made it my mission to send recipes to dear friends who could send me nutrient-dense snacks to simply do that . . . snack on. Snacks like my granola, zucchini bread, or avocado chocolate pudding when I couldn't chew food.

My message is, if you can't pronounce the ingredients, chances are your body probably can't break them down as easily. It is likely processed.

I am sharing recipes I shared live on my many *Clean Eating* segments on my show at FOX 7. Some were made by my amazing vegan chef, Lisa Buenaventura Rice, who taught me so much. My goal was and still is to help people prepare their bodies for illness and transform their diets. I hope you love them as much as I do.

People often ask, "Did you clean up your diet after you were diagnosed with cancer?"

I look at them and say, "Uhh, no. It was clean before. Before cancer I was gluten-free, diary-free, sugar-free, and caffeine-free, and I loved taking unhealthy meals and converting them into amazing clean meals for all to love." Ask anyone in the FOX 7 newsroom about how disciplined I was. Each day, bakeries and restaurants would drop off snacks from cupcakes to brownies, sub sandwiches and other treats to promote their next best items, and each time my colleagues would say, "Just eat it. Just cheat one time!" and they never got me to budge unless . . . it was a clean-eating recipe like a date-sweetened dessert or a meal with a healthy food swap.

For as long as I can remember, I have been living 75 to 80 percent plant-based, but this year I have decided, after a discussion with my Johns Hopkins cardiologist, that I needed to take my diet up another notch and go 100 percent plant-based and add in intermittent fasting or basically a compressed eating schedule of eating in either a six or eight-hour window each day. I'm basically cutting out all foods that can cause inflammation in my body and create an inflammatory response.

Here is why.

In June of 2020, my Johns Hopkins leukemia oncologist told me, "If I knew in 2014, what I know today, we would have never given you your sister's bone marrow." He went on to say, "We gave you, through your new DNA and transplant, a genetic marker named CHIP (clonal hematopoiesis of indeterminate potential) which has put a lot of stress on your body and put you into an inflammatory state. Now we know why you have suffered so much with everything from severe graft vs host disease from your transplant to constant recurring shingles, hives, and long- term health issues to a larger extent than most patients who survive."

He added, "The problem with CHIP is that it means you will not just have heart disease and risk of stroke and coronary heart disease, but you are now ten times more likely to develop a blood cancer or disorder like the very one you already fought." Dr. Levis told me that now bone-marrow transplant donors are screened for CHIP and are disqualified if they carry the marker. In my interpretation, consider it like the BRCA gene for breast cancer, except in this case you can't run and get another transplant to avoid another cancer because you already had one.

The bottom line is, as Dr. Levis told me as I sat and sobbed in his office, "Your sister gave you the gift of time. How much and what can happen next to you, we don't know. But you now have a cancer predisposition gene and breast cancer may not be your last to fight."

The good news is my medical team of doctors, including oncologists, cardiologists, neurologists, gastroenterologists, immunologists, ophthalmologists, psychologists, and last but not least a team of infectious disease doctors, all agree that I have continued to defy the odds and that my commitment to my clean diet, nonstop exercise and a lifestyle that focuses on meditation while eliminating stress is why they believe I'm still standing.

Going plant-based and removing any chance of added inflammation in my body can potentially save my life. It can make an impact on yours, too. You don't have to go 100 percent plant-based but you can start with a few small steps that can lead to big changes, even if it's one day a week or one meal a week.

I hope my story, my ArmorUp for LIFE® movement, and my message on how you can "Become your own Hero" by getting prepared so you can present well will become your mantra so you too can defy the odds and position yourself to prevail no matter what you might face.

NUTRIENT-DENSE HOMEMADE GRANOLA

This is one of my favorites and was a delicious snacking treat when I was fighting leukemia. I didn't have an appetite and I was nauseous, but I knew I needed nutrients. This is a tasty nutrient-dense snack that you can make for yourself at home or make for someone battling cancer. This recipe is great. You can customize to your liking and add more toppings as you go.

Ingredients

- 4 1/2 cups rolled oats (not quick-cooking)
- 1 1/3 cup flaked coconut (unsweetened)
- 1 heaping cup sliced almonds
- 1 heaping cup raw unsalted sunflower seeds
- 3/4 cup coarsely chopped raw almonds or whole raw almonds or any other nuts you love!
- 1-2 Tbsp. or more coconut sugar, monk fruit sugar, or date sweetener
- 1/3 cup coconut oil, liquid (warm in pan to melt), or 1/3 cup grapeseed oil
- 1 cup brown rice syrup (can also use 1/2 maple syrup, 1/2 brown rice syrup)
- 1/3 cup water
- 1 Tbsp. alcohol-free vanilla extract
- Optional other items to consider adding AFTER you cook the granola:

- o 1/3 cup of dried cranberries or dried cherries
- o 1/3 cup of dried apricots
- o 1/3 cup of golden raisins
- o 1/3 cup of carob chips or stevia-sweetened chips

Cooking Instructions

- Preheat oven to 325 degrees.
- Mix dry ingredients in bowl.
- Melt coconut oil in saucepan and whisk in syrup, water, and vanilla.
- Stir wet ingredients into dry until combined.
- Spread mixture evenly on cookie sheet with sides. Bake 10 minutes at 325 degrees, then stir and then bake 10 minutes more. Stir every ten minutes until golden brown (2-3 times, most likely).
- Let cool on cookie sheet
- Once cool, break apart into chunks and mix in optional items.

AVOCADO CHOCOLATE MOUSSE

This is another amazing recipe. You will have no idea you are eating a nutrient-dense dessert and neither will anyone you share this dessert with.

Ingredients

- 2 avocados (ripe like you would need for guacamole, ready to eat)
- 1/2 cup 100% cacao (this is the real deal, not cocoa powder)
- 1/3 cup honey (or natural sweetener like maple syrup, coconut sugar, monk fruit sugar, or stevia)
- 1/2 cup almond/cashew or coconut milk
- 1/2 tsp. vanilla

Instructions

- Blend all ingredients.
- Top with a few tiny morsels of chocolate. (*I love the stevia sweetened chips.*)
- (Optional) Add in protein powder and/or collagen peptides to give this a protein boost.

GLUTEN-FREE (ALMOND FLOUR) CHOCOLATE MUFFINS

This is another great snack to nibble on. Try adding the avocado chocolate mousse as an icing with a little coconut whipped topping (recipe to follow) and you are in business!

Ingredients

- 1 tsp. melted butter, ghee or coconut oil
- 4 eggs
- 1/2 cup honey
- 1 tsp. vanilla extract
- 1 cup (4 ounces) almond flour
- 1/2 cup unsweetened cacao powder
- 1/2 tsp. kosher salt
- 1/2 tsp. baking soda

Instructions

- Spray a 12-cup muffin pan with cooking spray. Mix all ingredients in a bowl. Pour into prepared pan.
- Bake 15 minutes at 325 degrees.
- Voila! Amazing muffins.

CITRUS VINAIGRETTE SALAD DRESSINGS

Ditch the bottled grocery-store bought dressings and make it yourself. This has six ingredients and you will love it! No preservatives, nothing artificial—just pure goodness. Top any salad you want, including kale salads.

Ingredients

- 1/2 cup white balsamic vinegar
- 1/2 cup olive oil
- 2 Tbsp. honey
- 1/3 cup fresh squeezed orange juice
- 1/2 tsp. red chili flakes (add more for a little kick)
- 1/2 tsp. oregano

Instructions

- Combine all ingredients in a small bowl or shaker bottle. Mix well.

This dressing is GREAT on any salad but my favorite is as a kale salad. The best part of adding this dressing to kale is that you can make this in advance and the kale salad will stay yummy for days. First, drizzle on a little olive oil. Massage the kale leaves to break them down a bit and soften them. Add cranberries and slivered almonds, and then top it all with the dressing. It is AMAZING.

KALE SALAD

Ingredients

- 1 bag of organic kale
- 1 Tbsp. olive oil
- 1/4 cup of dried cranberries
- 1/4 cup of slivered almonds
- Citrus Vinaigrette Salad Dressing (above)

Instructions

- Wash kale; put in medium-sized bowl.
- Massage the olive oil into the kale with your hands to break down the leaves and soften them.
- Sprinkle on cranberries and almonds.
- Add the dressing on top and mix well. Voila—it's amazing and stores well in the fridge for days!

FIG DRESSING

Ingredients

- 1/4 cup balsamic vinegar
- 1 Tbsp. apple cider vinegar, white vinegar, or fresh lemon juice
- 2 Tbsp. fig fruit spread
- 1/4 cup olive oil
- 1 Tbsp. Tamari
- Fresh cracked black pepper to taste

CHICKPEA BURGERS

Ingredients

- 1 - 2 Tbsp. olive oil
- 1 large white or yellow onion, diced
- 2 garlic gloves, minced
- 2 scallions, sliced
- 1 tsp. sea salt
- 1/2 tsp. black pepper
- 1 1/2 tsp. cumin
- 1 1/2 tsp. coriander
- 1/2 tsp. smoked paprika
- 3 cups chickpeas
- 1/8 cup garbanzo bean flour, almond flour, or oat flour

Instructions

- Heat oil in a sauté pan over medium heat, then add the chopped onion, garlic and sauté until soft.
- Add scallions, salt, pepper, cumin, coriander, and paprika and cook a few minutes more until fragrant and scallions are wilted. Remove from heat.
- In a medium bowl, mash chickpeas until broken down a bit, but still chunky (leave some whole).
- Add the cooked onion mixture to the chickpeas and mix thoroughly. Add the flour.
- Using a half-cup measure, form burger-sized shapes from the mixture and place on an oiled baking dish or cookie sheet.

- Spray tops of the burgers lightly with olive oil. Bake for approximately 30 minutes at 400 degrees.

Variations

- Mexican flair: Add chopped cilantro, a chopped banana pepper, and minced jalapeño.
- Italian flair: Leave out cumin, coriander and paprika, and substitute 1/4 tsp. each of dried basil, thyme, and oregano (or chopped fresh basil, thyme and oregano).

DAIRY-FREE RECIPES

Vegan "Raw" Queso

You can't live in Texas and not have tacos as part of your diet. Here is a great vegan recipe that has all the "fix-ins" to make your heart happy and it is packed with nutrients.

Ingredients

- 2 medium-sized red bell peppers, seeded and chopped
- 1 heaping cup raw cashews/cashew pieces, soaked (2 hours of soaking or more, the longer the better for a creamy texture)
- 2 cloves garlic
- Juice of 1 small lime (about 1/8 cup)
- 1 Tbsp. apple cider vinegar
- 1 Tbsp. olive oil
- 1 tsp. sea salt
- 1/2 tsp. ground cumin
- 1/2 cup nutritional yeast

Instructions

- Put everything in a blender (peppers on bottom) and blend until smooth, scraping down sides as needed. Great as a dip for chips and great on beans, tacos, and enchiladas.

Vegan "Raw" Tacos

Taco "Meat" Ingredients

- 3 cups walnuts
- 1/3 cup Tamari/Soy sauce or Coconut Liquid Aminos
- 1 tsp. coriander
- 1 tsp. cumin

Instructions

- Grind walnuts fine in food processor, mix in bowl with seasonings.

Salsa (In bowl, mix)

- 3 cups chopped grape, cherry or Roma tomatoes or combination
- 1/4 medium white onion chopped small (about 1/2 cup), or 1/2 cup chopped green onion
- 1 red bell pepper, chopped small
- 1/2 tsp. sea salt
- 1 cup roughly chopped cilantro leaves

In blender or Magic Bullet

- 1 large lime juiced (about 1/4 cup)
- 1/2 cup chopped unsalted and unseasoned sun-dried tomatoes
- 1/8 cup olive oil
- 2 cloves garlic

- 1 tsp. cumin
- optional: 1/8 tsp. habanero pepper or 1/4 tsp. cayenne pepper or 1 fresh jalapeño seeded and minced

Instructions

- Blend well and stir into tomato mixture.
- Fresh avocado, sliced for garnish.
- Assemble: lay out collard leaf, spread taco filling lengthwise, first layer walnut meat, second layer salsa, third layer fresh avocado, finish with dollop of queso.

Variations

- Use romaine lettuce leaves instead of collards
- Use store-bought fresh salsa or *pico de gallo* instead of recipe.

DESSERTS

Pumpkin Crumb-Cake Muffin

Ingredients

- 3 egg whites
- 1 cup organic pumpkin puree
- 1/3 organic coconut milk (full fat)
- 1 1/8 tsp. vanilla extract
- 2 1/2 Tbsp. maple syrup
- 6 dates (pitted, softened in warm water, and pureed), or 1/3 cup coconut or monk fruit sugar
- 2 cups almond flour
- 1/4 cup arrowroot flour or tapioca starch
- 1 Tbsp. coconut flour
- 1/8 tsp. turmeric
- 1 Tbsp. pumpkin pie spice
- 3/4 tsp. cinnamon
- 1 tsp. baking soda

Crumb topping

- 1/2 cup almond flour
- 2 Tbsp. coconut oil, melted
- 1 tsp. pumpkin pie spice
- 1/3 cup coconut sugar (or monk fruit sugar)

Instructions

- Preheat oven to 350 degrees. Spray a 12-cup muffin pan with cooking spray.
- Mix the egg, pumpkin puree, coconut milk, vanilla, and maple syrup in one bowl and set aside.
- In a separate bowl, take the softened soaked dates and drain the water. Put them in a Vitamix or blender and puree.
- Add dates to the egg mixture and mix.
- In a separate bowl, mix the dry ingredients (flours, turmeric, pumpkin pie spice, cinnamon, and baking soda).
- Add dry ingredients to the wet ingredients and mix.
- Spoon into a muffin pan. Top each muffin with a teaspoon of crumb topping.
- Bake 35-40 minutes.

Keto Key Lime Pie

Ingredients

- 1 can of coconut cream (only use the creamy part. I love the Trader Joe's brand)
- 1/2 cup of lime juice (fresh squeezed is best)
- 1 cup softened cashews (soak in warm water for 2 hours and drain)
- 1/2 cup coconut sugar or monk fruit sugar

Instructions

- Mix all ingredients in a Vitamix or high-powered blender.

Ingredients (Pie Crust)

- 1 cup coconut flour
- 1 tsp. cinnamon
- 1 tsp. nutmeg
- 1 tsp. coconut oil
- 2 Tbsp. coconut sugar

Instructions

- Mix together. Spray a small pie pan.
- Press the pie crust into the pan with your thumbs until the pan is covered.
- Pour the key lime mix into pan; put in the fridge for a few hours and then enjoy!!

Cinnamon "Cookie Dough" Balls

Ingredients

- 1/2 cup raw cashews
- 2 Tbsp. hemp seeds
- 1/8 tsp. sea salt
- 1 tsp. cinnamon
- 3/4 cup rolled oats
- 1 cup pitted dates
- 1/2 tsp. vanilla
- 2 Tbsp. shredded unsweetened coconut
- 1-2 Tbsp. miniature non-dairy chocolate chips

Instructions

In a food processor, add the cashews, hemp seeds, salt, cinnamon, and oats and grind until crumbly. Add the dates and vanilla, and spin again for a minute or more. When the mixture begins to clump and stick, add the coconut and chocolate chips and process again. Continue to process until dough forms a ball on the blade. Stop the machine and remove the dough. If making balls: Take small scoops of the dough (a couple teaspoons each) and roll in your hands. Repeat until you have rolled all of the dough. Refrigerate for an hour or more until chilled. Can also be pressed into a pan to make bars.

Sumptuous Lemon Bar Balls

Ingredients

- 1 cup raw cashews
- 1/2 cup raw almonds
- 2 lemons, juiced and zested (separate juice from zest)
- 10 - 12 medjool dates, pits removed
- Garnish: 1/2-3/4 cups shredded coconut

Instructions

Blend nuts and zest in the processor until broken down a bit. Add dates and juice and process until a smooth mass forms. Roll walnut-sized balls in your palms. If desired, roll each ball in coconut (can also be made into bars).

Chill in fridge and enjoy!

Decadent Raw Vegan Chocolate truffles

Ingredients

- 1 - 2 cups medjool dates, pits removed
- 1 - 2 cups raw Brazil nuts
- 1 vanilla bean, scraped, or 1/2 tsp. alcohol-free vanilla
- 1/4 cup (or more) raw cacao powder or unsweetened cocoa powder
- Pinch or two of Himalayan salt
- Optional garnish: 1/2 cup or more cacao or cocoa powder or 1/2 cup shredded coconut

Instructions

Blend dates, Brazil nuts, and vanilla in food processor until dough clumps into a thick mass (kind of like Play-doh). Roll walnut-sized balls in your hands (it will get very oily from the nuts). Roll each ball in cacao/cocoa powder (1/2 cup may not be enough, so be prepared to add more as you go along). Take half the balls you've rolled in the powder and roll in the coconut.

Chill in fridge and enjoy!

COCONUT CASHEW "WHIPPED TOPPING"

Ingredients

- 1 cup raw cashews or cashew pieces, soaked overnight and drained
- 1 12 or 14 oz. can coconut cream - I use Trader Joe's extra thick and rich (if you can't get the coconut cream, use full fat coconut milk and use less water)
- 1 vanilla bean, scraped, or 1 Tbsp. vanilla
- 3 Tbsp. maple syrup
- Pinch of good sea salt
- Water as needed for blending (up to 3/4 cup if using coconut cream)

Instructions

Blend everything until smooth, pour into glass or ceramic dish, cover, and chill for several hours or overnight. The mixture will thicken while it sits. Stir before serving.

Herbed Cashew Cheese

Ingredients

- 2 cups raw cashews or cashew pieces, soaked for at least 2 hours to overnight and drained
- 2/3 cup water
- Juice of 1/2 lemon (about 2 tablespoons)
- 1/8 cup nutritional yeast

- 1/4 tsp. garlic powder
- 1/4 tsp. onion powder
- 1/2 tsp. sea salt
- 2 capsules probiotics (empty into blender and discard capsules) (I used PB 8 but you can use whatever brand you've got, or skip this if you don't have any and it will turn out fine!)
- 2 scallions or green onions, white and part of green, minced
- 1 small shallot, minced
- 2 -3 Tbsp. of flat leaf parsley, chopped small

Instructions

- Blend nuts, water, lemon juice, yeast, garlic powder, sea salt, and probiotics (if using) until smooth.
- Transfer to bowl and stir in remaining ingredients.
- Chill in fridge at least an hour before serving. Great on crackers, crostini, sliced baguette, crudités, toasted bagels, and as a sandwich spread.

Variations

Try adding other fresh herbs like tarragon, basil and thyme, or cilantro and mint, or mix in olives or capers. Change it up to match your other dishes!

Tofu Sour Cream

Ingredients

- 1 package extra-firm silken tofu
- 1 1/2 Tbsp. umeboshi vinegar
- 1 Tbsp. olive oil
- 1 tsp. mustard powder
- 1/4 tsp. garlic powder
- 1 tsp. dried dill or 2 Tbsp. chopped fresh

Instructions

Blend everything but dill in food processor. Transfer to bowl and stir in dill. Chill until ready to serve.

OYSTER MUSHROOMS

https://www.mskcc.org/cancer-care/integrative-medicine/herbs/oyster-mushroom

Oyster mushrooms are an edible fungus found widely in North America and Europe. They are used in traditional medicine to treat infections, hyperlipidemia, diabetes, and cancer. According to Sloan Kettering Hospital, laboratory experiments have shown that *oyster mushrooms* have anti-tumor, anti-fungal, and cholesterol-lowering properties.

They are my new favorite!

Here are a few recipes to try.

Vegan "Fajita" Oyster Mushroom Sauté

Ingredients

- 3 Tbsp. oil (I prefer avocado oil)
- 1 small red bell pepper, sliced
- 1 small yellow bell pepper, sliced
- 1 red onion, sliced (yellow sweet onions work great too!)
- 2 king oyster mushrooms, thinly sliced
- ¼ tsp. each cumin, chili powder, oregano and salt
- Fajita toppings (cheese, salsa, sour cream, avocado, cilantro, etc.)
- Tortillas or cauliflower rice

Instructions

- Heat 1 Tbsp. of oil in a sauce pan, add peppers and onion. Cook until softened, and sauté about 10 minutes. Remove to a plate.
- Add remaining 2 Tbsp. canola oil, then mushrooms. Cook until caramelized, stirring occasionally, about 15 minutes.
- Add spices and salt, cook another 3 minutes.
- Serve mushrooms with peppers and onion either in a tortilla or on a bed of cauliflower rice to keep it low carb. Top with salsa, fresh cilantro, avocado and non-dairy cheese. Try topping this with my non-dairy vegan queso!

Pan Fried Oyster Mushrooms

Ingredients

- 2 Tbsp. olive oil
- 12 ounces oyster mushrooms, cut into evenly sized pieces
- 3 garlic cloves, smashed
- 5 sprigs of thyme
- 2 Tbsp. butter or ghee
- sea salt and black pepper to taste

Instructions

- Heat the olive oil in a large, heavy skillet over medium high heat.
- Spread the mushrooms out in a single layer in the pan. Cook undisturbed for 3-5 minutes until they start to brown.

- Stir the mushrooms and cook for another 3-5 minutes until browned all over.
- Add the garlic, thyme, and butter/ghee to the skillet and reduce the heat to low. Cook for another 5-6 minutes, spooning the ghee/butter over the mushrooms until they are dark brown and slightly crispy.
- Remove the thyme springs and season the mushrooms with salt and pepper to taste. Enjoy!

Spicy Oyster Mushroom Stir-Fry

Ingredients

- 1 lb. oyster mushrooms
- 5 Tbsp. oil of your choice (I like high heat oils like avocado oil, which also contains healthy fat) plus it's a good fat
- 5 long hot peppers (red or green)
- 4-6 slices of ginger
- 4-6 cloves of sliced garlic (add more if you like a big garlic taste)
- 1/2 tsp. coconut sugar
- 1 Tbsp. spicy bean sauce
- 2 Tbsp. of soy sauce or coconut aminos for added benefit
- Green onions
- Scallions (you can use these if you are skipping the hot peppers and need a little more flavor)

Instructions

- Cut the mushrooms in half lengthwise.
- Heat the oil in a wok over high heat. Place mushrooms in pan cut side down.
- Fry the mushrooms lightly until tender and set aside.
- Reduce the heat, add ginger and then gradually add garlic. After one minute add the bean sauce.
- Add mushrooms back to the wok, along with the light soy sauce or coconut aminos and 1/2 tsp. of coconut sugar (this is lower glycemic than real sugar and better for you!)
- Stir fry everything, and then serve over cauliflower rice or gluten-free noodles.

PALEO CHINESE CASHEW CHICKEN

Ingredients

- 2 lbs. chicken (or one pack of firm tofu)
- 2 Ttbsp. sesame oil
- 1/2 cup of coconut aminos
- 3 Tbsp. ketchup (no-sugar-added ketchup is best)
- 3 Tbsp. rice vinegar
- 1 Tbsp. coconut sugar
- 1 Tbsp. honey
- 1 Tbsp. minced garlic
- 1 1/4 Tbsp. minced ginger
- 2 Tbsp. arrowroot flour
- 1/2 tsp. red pepper flakes
- 1/4 tsp. salt
- 1/4 tsp. pepper
- 2 Tbsp. water
- 1 cup slightly softened cashews
- Broccoli

Instructions

- This is a great Instant Pot meal but if you are using tofu you should not use the instant pot. Instead, I recommend that you grill your tofu, mix the sauce separately, and then mix on the stove.
- If you don't like the broccoli too soft then I recommend steaming it separately and then topping the meal with it.

If you are using the Instant Pot:

- Brown the meat in the sesame oil by using the sauté button.
- Mix the remaining ingredients in a separate bowl (minus the arrowroot flour and cashews) and set aside.
- Once the meat is brown, pour the sauce over the chicken.
- Set the Instant Pot to 10 minutes and let it cook.
- In a separate bowl mix the 2 Tbsp. of arrowroot flour with 1 Tbsp. of water.
- Once it is finished, quickly stir in your flour mixture to thicken it. Then add your cashews, pour over cauliflower rice, and ENJOY!

CAULIFLOWER

Cauliflower Latkes

These are amazing and like potato pancakes, but with cauliflower.

Ingredients

- ½ head of cauliflower (or fresh cauliflower rice)
- ½ cup of scallions, thinly sliced
- 1 Tbsp. of golden flaxseed meal, or you can swap for 2 Tbsp. of gluten-free flour
- 2 Eggs (or egg replacer-you can also use flax for this by sitting flax in water and letting it thicken. This works as a great binder)
- 2 Tbsp. of nutritional yeast
- 1 ½ tsp. of Salt
- ½ tsp. of Pepper
- 1/2 cup of non-dairy shredded cheese or regular cheddar

Dipping sauce

Ingredients

- 3 Tbsp. vegan mayo
- 1 Tbsp. chili sauce

Instructions

- Separate the cauliflower into florets and steam.
- Combine the flax meal and water. Place into the refrigerator until ready to use.

- Drain any condensation by placing the florets onto paper towels.
- Put in food processor but don't over-process. You want the cauliflower broken up, not creamy.
- Combine all of the dry ingredients with a whisk.
- Add the flax mixture and processed cauliflower pieces, stirring well to combine. The mixture will still be very moist.
- Preheat a large skillet on medium-high heat (or bake in oven or air fryer).
- Add the oil and put spoonfuls down to brown on each side, much like you would with a pancake.
- Continue cooking until browned on both sides.
- Transfer to paper towels, pat dry and drop with dipping sauce! ENJOY!

Crispy Buffalo Cauliflower Wings

Ingredients

- 1 head cauliflower
- 1 cup almond or coconut flour
- 1 cup dairy-free milk/water
- 1 cup gluten-free bread crumbs
- 1 Tbsp. garlic powder
- 1 tsp. smoked paprika
- 1/2 tsp. salt
- 1 cup buffalo sauce
- 1 Tbsp. ghee or butter

Instructions

- First, preheat oven to 450 F or I LOVE using my air fryer!
- Line a baking sheet with parchment paper.
- Rinse and cut cauliflower into bite-sized pieces. Pat dry.
- In a large bowl, combine the flour and milk. Whisk until combined.
- In another large bowl, combine the bread crumbs, garlic powder, smoked paprika, and salt.
- Drip each cauliflower floret into the (milk/flour) batter and coat evenly.
- Then dip the floret into the dry bowl with bread crumbs.
- Next, lay the florets on the baking sheet.
- Bake for 10 minutes.
- Flip. Then bake the other side for another 10 minutes.
- While the cauliflower is baking, grab a small saucepan, put it on low heat and add the buffalo sauce and butter. Stir until butter has melted.
- Coat the wings with the buffalo sauce. Then, add them back onto the baking sheet.
- Bake for another 10 minutes. Flip. Then bake the other side for another 10 minutes.

SWEET POTATO FRIES AND DIPPING SAUCE

Ingredients

- 4 Sweet Potatoes
- Olive Oil spray (I love Trader Joe's brand. Its only ingredient is olive oil)
- Salt, pepper, garlic powder to sprinkle on (to taste)
- 1/4 cup spicy brown mustard (Trader Joe's brand is the best)
- 2 Tbsp. honey

Instructions

- Cut sweet potatoes in long strips like fries.
- Spray them with olive oil spray.
- Sprinkle on salt, pepper, garlic powder to your liking
- Put in the air fryer for 20 min (but toss every 5 minutes) until crispy. You can also bake in the oven on 400 F.

Dipping sauce

- Mix the spicy mustard and the honey and VIOLA! It's amazing.
- You might even like to use this dip for other yummy meals.

INDIAN CURRY (USING MANY SPICES!)

Ingredients

- 2 Tbsp. avocado or olive oil
- 1 large yellow onion, finely diced
- 2-3 inch piece of fresh ginger, minced
- 3 medium cloves garlic, minced
- 1 Tbsp. ground coriander
- 1-1/2 tsp. ground cumin
- 3/4 tsp. ground turmeric
- 1/2 tsp. Cayenne pepper
- 1/8 tsp. cinnamon or a cinnamon stick
- 2 tomatoes (pureed in the blender) or 4 ounces tomato sauce
- 2 cups lower-salt chicken broth or vegetable broth
- 1 cup light coconut milk
- 1 small cauliflower, broken into pieces
- 1 lb. sweet potatoes, cut into cubes
- 2 large carrots, peeled and cut into 1/2-inch-thick rounds (about 1 cup)
- One 15-1/2-oz. can chickpeas, drained and rinsed
- 4 oz. baby spinach (about 4 lightly packed cups)
- 2 Tbsp. fresh lime juice
- 1 tsp. finely grated lime zest
- 2 Tbsp. chopped fresh cilantro

Instructions

I love my Instant Pot. This can be easily cooked in there.

- Put it in the sauté mode, add the onions and oil to cook for about 5 minutes.
- Add your garlic, ginger and keep stirring. Add in the remainder of the spices (coriander, cumin, turmeric, cinnamon and Cayenne).
- Add the tomato sauce and let it sauté for a few more minutes.
- Add the broth, coconut milk, cinnamon and a dash of salt and pepper
- Toss in your cauliflower, sweet potatoes, tomatoes, and carrots, chickpeas, spinach, lime juice, and zest;
- Cook for 10 minutes on high pressure, garnish with cilantro, and ENJOY!
- **If you want to add chicken to this recipe you can always brown the chicken before you start and then add it back in when it is time to start the pressure cook. Either way, it is amazing.

CONGEE

When I would call my acupuncturist, Kirsten Karchmer, for any problem, her answer was always, "Are you eating your congee?"

In Chinese medicine, congee is used to promote good health, harmonize digestion and supplement the blood. Congee is believed to relieve inflammation and nourishes the immune system. There are countless ways to enjoy congee, including plain, with fruit, or as a meal.

Ingredients

- 1 cup brown rice
- 8 cups water
- Add-ins, such as dried apricots, cinnamon, nutmeg, ginger, or other spices
- Nuts (how much for a serving?)

Cook in the Instant Pot or a slow cooker for 15 minutes. When it is finished, add nuts on top. I ate this daily when doing acupuncture for fertility to have our son Gabriel, and still do in various varieties.

For a lunch or dinner meal, you can do so much. You can first sauté onions, garlic, ginger and mushrooms and then start your congee and add to it with scallions.

DRINKS

Cold pressed juices are great for you. My favorite is celery juice with a little bit of lemon in it. It's a great detox and immune booster. But since I'm Cuban I can't help but share this clean drinking mojito.

Ingredients

- 1 1/2 cups coconut water
- 1 Tbsp. fresh lime juice
- 1 cup spinach
- 1/2 avocado
- 1/3 cup nuts (cashews or macadamia)
- Handful of mint leaves
- 1/2 tsp. vanilla extract or powder
- 1/8 tsp. minced ginger
- 1 scoop of collagen peptides
- 2 Tbsp. of honey or 5-6 drops of stevia

Instructions

- There are many options for your liquid. Swap the coconut water with just water if you prefer. To add back in the coconut flavor, just add a 1/2 tsp. of coconut oil. You can also swap and use green tea.
- Put all the ingredients in a high-powered blender; pour into a glass, top with more mint, and you are ready to go!

Golden Milk

This is a yummy drink and a great way to end your day. In Ayurvedic medicine it is believed to be an immune-boosting drink because of its anti-inflammatory properties.

Ingredients

- 1/2 cups light coconut milk
- 1 1/2 cups unsweetened almond milk
- 1 1/2 tsp. ground turmeric
- 1/4 tsp. ground ginger
- 1/4 tsp. cinnamon (optional - not all recipes use the cinnamon)
- 1/4 tsp. vanilla (optional - not all recipes use this ingredient)
- Pinch cardamom
- 1 Tbsp. coconut oil
- 1 pinch black pepper (this helps with digestion of turmeric)
- Sweetener of choice (maple syrup, coconut sugar, or stevia) to taste

Instructions

- Put all ingredients in a small saucepan. Heat for 4 minutes. Turn off heat and taste to adjust flavor. Add more sweetener to taste or more turmeric or ginger for intense spice + flavor.
- Serve immediately.

FOOD FUN FACTS

- Dates are high in potassium and loaded with minerals. They are also full of antioxidants. They are a great whole food sweetener and are actually low on the glycemic index. Coupled with the healthy fats from raw nuts, they are great for sustained energy.

- Raw hemp seeds are a healthy source of protein (3 Tablespoons have 11 grams of protein). They are high in omega fatty acids, which make them great for fighting inflammation, as well as great for the skin and hair. Hemp seeds are also high in antioxidants.

- Walnuts are not only good for the heart, but they are great for the brain, especially short-term memory. They are high in Omega-3 fatty acids and vitamin E, which in studies have proven to lower the risk of Alzheimer's.

- Avocados are high in potassium and vitamins (C,A,K,B) and healthy fats (omega 3), good for inflammation, and a great brain food!

- Nuts and seeds are excellent sources of protein for vegans and vegetarians. Ground and seasoned and used as meat substitutes, they also provide great texture (and of course fiber).

- Walnuts and cashews are both healthy sources of unsaturated fats, minerals, and antioxidants. They are both good sources of vitamin E.

- Walnuts have proven to help reduce bad cholesterol (LDL). They are also rich in alpha linolenic acid which helps protect the heart during times of acute stress.

Because they are a good source of vitamin E and also contain folate (a B vitamin), they are good for the brain, especially short-term memory!

- Cashews are a good source of magnesium, which helps balance potassium levels. Low magnesium levels can raise blood pressure. Cashews are also a good source of vitamin E.
- Nutritional Yeast is a good source of protein and is an umami-tasting condiment wildly popular with vegans because it helps provide a cheesy flavor and texture to nut-based cheese and sauce recipes. Because of the way it is grown (it's basically a healthy bacteria grown in molasses), it is a good source of (and often fortified with) B vitamins which many vegans and vegetarians lack.

Epilogue

HOMECOMING.
HOME SWEET HOME.
NOT HOME, HOME.

I don't know what it feels like to walk out of prison after incarceration, but I think I came close to it when I got home from the hospital. It was a Christmas Day miracle.

I wanted lights up.

I wanted the house to look like a fairy tale.

I wanted to have it like a made-for-television movie because it sure felt like one.

I wanted to run into my son's arms.

And . . . I did.

FINALLY.

I was home. Not "home" home like I had feared.

I held my son.

I didn't want to get up.

Then I couldn't wait to take a damn shower and feel ALL of the water hit every inch of my body. It had been an entire year since I'd had that freedom. I was used to taking showers with my arm in a bag and my chest covered in plastic to protect my Hickman catheter so water wouldn't get inside. I couldn't let the water hit my chest so I would lean in or halfway lean out of the shower. My entire body didn't get covered by water in a shower for a year. After holding my son and hugging him all day long, the first thing I did once he went to sleep was stand in my shower, look up at the water, let it hit my face, and say, "AHHHHHHH FREEDOM!" out loud. Freedom to relax and take a shower. Freedom to let the water fall freely. Freedom to bathe myself and feel so independent. Woo hoo! It felt so damn good. So many things we take for granted. A real shower was one of them.

I couldn't wait to sleep through the night without having to wake up for medications. I couldn't wait to walk outside without an IV attached to my arm and pushing a pole on wheels. I couldn't wait to smell fresh air. I couldn't wait to walk through a grocery store and pick out my own food. The list goes on and on . . . and included smelling the fresh air and feeling free. I couldn't wait for the smell of freedom.

Free to make cookies with my son despite my exhaustion.

Free to hug again after we disinfect.

Free to make more memories.

Free to live my life again, or live the new one I was given.

I knew the old one was gone.

And for that, I was also very scared.

I knew I wasn't free from worry. I knew I still had a 25-percent chance of seeing Gabriel reach seven. I knew it took five years for the transplant to officially "work." I was scared of what would happen if something happened and now, I'm so far from my oncologist. I knew only my Hopkins team understood my transplant, and any pop-up problems had to be handled there. It was not down the street. An hour and a half each way. I had done that drive alone. I had no choice. We needed health insurance. My husband needed to work. I was challenged. I overcame it.

While everyone around me was celebrating my win, I was fully aware of the stats and I knew in my heart to clap quietly. Yes, I have come far. But I know you don't win leukemia and a bone-marrow transplant until you survive five years. I know that perfectly well. I've witnessed it. And even while embracing being reunited with my son and finally being all under one roof, I knew it wasn't over. As I tried to get reintroduced with my world and get reacquainted with my son, I struggled. Who was I? I found myself in a mind and body I barely recognized.

I quickly learned the fight doesn't end after that last drip of chemo. In fact, a whole new fight and struggle was about to begin. Survivorship. A world where you are given a new chance at life but no tools to navigate the system. And there I was, reunited with my son. I lost my hair, my DNA, my identity, my career. I kept asking myself, "Do I make memories in case I die, or resumes in case I live?"

It was like the scene from *Alice in Wonderland* where Alice says, "I wonder if I've been changed in the night. Let me think. Was I the same when I got up this morning? I almost think I can remember feeling a little different. But I'm not the same, the next question is, who in the world am I? Ah, that's a great puzzle."

We may have all evolved in our personal and professional lives while going through the pandemic. Maybe you know your DNA and you didn't battle leukemia but you aren't the person you were when this pandemic started. My message to you is, you have the chance TODAY to go beyond the mask and "Become your own HERO." To make choices to change how you live your life. To make decisions that will determine how well you are prepared for any illnesses like COVID, cancer, or heart disease.

You can start today by reducing the stress in your life, taking action to limit the behaviors that add inflammation to your life. I'm either your coach or your cautionary tale.

Choose one.

PREPARE-PRESENT-PREVAIL. ®

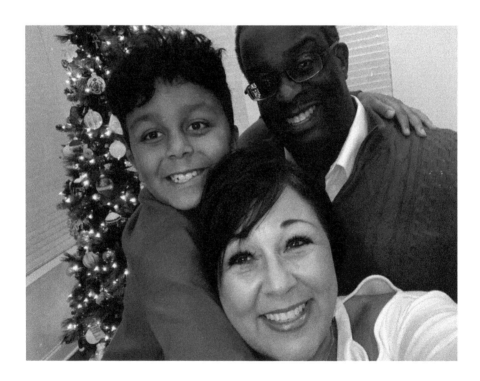

Call to Action

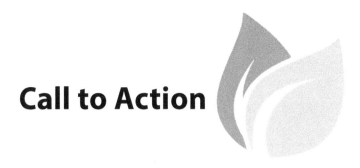

It is time to make patients POSSIBLE.

My 3P protocol can save lives and make more patients possible.

Rather than asking patients to beat the odds, it is time we change the odds.

I'm calling on leaders, decision makers, academia and others in Pharma and Biotech to think outside the box and allocate funding not just when we fall ill but help us, including those in the brown and Black communities, better *present* once we do. This requires funding in "risk reduction" efforts not just clinical trial strategies. The time to fund PREHAB is now.

It's a win-win for patients and your latest innovation.

The longer we can stay in the game the more of your latest innovation and treatment we can handle.

While I am thrilled that we are finally having the conversation about *how* to increase diversity in clinical trials, build trust in our communities, remove barriers such as costs, transportation and childcare, and revise clinical trial strategies and research design that will broaden the eligibility criteria to allow more minorities into clinical trials, this is *not* enough.

We Need a Multi-tiered Approach

Yes, addressing these issues is long overdue. I'm directly impacted by this lack of diversity. Millions of others are too. I've missed many opportunities to enroll in trials due to barriers and lack of patient centric messaging to help me understand why trials were for me.

But we would be negligent if we didn't look deeper at this issue and ask *why*.

Why do we have to broaden the eligibility criteria in order to increase diversity in clinical trials? Because typically clinical trial criteria limits patients who have underlying health conditions and excludes them from trials.

Who has underlying health conditions at disproportionate rates? Communities of color. Studies show we don't present well compared to whites at times of illness. Communities of color present with many underlying health conditions and are disproportionately affected by hypertension, obesity and diabetes. Even worse, in many cases, these underlying problems are shown to be untreated.

Why are we not looking at the elephant in the room and the bigger problem when we have *these* conversations? We need to be out in our communities reducing the risk for underlying health conditions and addressing risk factors. Those in the brown and black communities already face health inequities in broad strokes that position them for lower patient outcomes.

I've been advocating for PREHAB long before COVID-19 but it may have taken a pandemic for many to see the reality of how showing up with underlying health conditions can be deadly and lower patient outcomes. Their genetic markers and social-economic barriers may set them up for failure with higher health risks but their zip codes should not.

Yes! How patients show up matters and we have a chance as a healthcare community to get involved early and radically change a patient's trajectory and chance of survival through education and early intervention.

As my world-renowned oncologist says, "Your treatment is directly related to how you present and what you can handle. We can't kill you trying to **save you.**"

Let's Address the Underlying Health Problems, Not Just Broaden the Rules to Help us Fit into Your New Criteria

If you help patients prepare better, they can present better at times of illness, and position them to prevail. They will be in the game longer to take your latest innovation. Patients want more. Patients deserve more. We are not just subjects. We are not just numbers and not just your N1s. We are whole patients with real life problems.

What I'm asking for is not impossible. We make it impossible when we stay in our lane.

When we ignore the whole patient, the baggage he or she might bring and how it might impact the next step and the course of treatment. We need collaboration with your innovation across the board.

Collaboration among care teams.

You Did it During Covid Successfully

You collaborated across the industry and created a vaccine in record time with goals and innovation. Let's take this energy and strategies and do it over and over again. I challenge you, our leaders and academia in healthcare, to look at your mission, your vision and what needs to happen.

How can we help patients PREPARE for illness so they can present better to you and —how can "we" collectively position them to "PREVAIL"— ArmorUp for LIFE®

At ArmorUp for LIFE, we envision a world where PREHAB is just as important as REHAB and when patients become ill the healthcare system is proactive in the approach to provide resources needed to treat the WHOLE patient, mentally and physically with equal access for all patients.

Every patient should have the chance to survive like I did.

Every patient should be possible.

CPSIA information can be obtained
at www.ICGtesting.com
Printed in the USA
BVHW020324270722
643094BV00002B/2

9 781737 061403